Health Insurance

Edited by Aida Isabel Tavares

Published in London, United Kingdom

Health Insurance
http://dx.doi.org/10.5772/intechopen.98015
Edited by Aida Isabel Tavares

Contributors
Ian Duncan, Samuel George Anarwat, Salisu Hassan, Maria Cristina G. Bautista, John Geyman, Aida Isabel Tavares, Tomoyuki Takura, Valentina Prevolnik Rupel, Tit Albreht, Marjeta Kuhar, Hasbullah Thabrany, Mutia Sayekti, Diriba Feyisa

First published in London, United Kingdom, 2022 by IntechOpen
IntechOpen is the global imprint of INTECHOPEN LIMITED, registered in England and Wales, registration number: 11086078, 5 Princes Gate Court, London, SW7 2QJ, United Kingdom

British Library Cataloguing-in-Publication Data
A catalogue record for this book is available from the British Library

Additional hard and PDF copies can be obtained from orders@intechopen.com

Health Insurance
Edited by Aida Isabel Tavares
p. cm.
Print ISBN 978-1-80355-870-7
Online ISBN 978-1-80355-871-4
eBook (PDF) ISBN 978-1-80355-872-1

For EU product safety concerns:
IN TECH d.o.o., Prolaz Marije Krucifikse Kozulić 3, 51000 Rijeka, Croatia,
info@intechopen.com or visit our website at intechopen.com.

Meet the editor

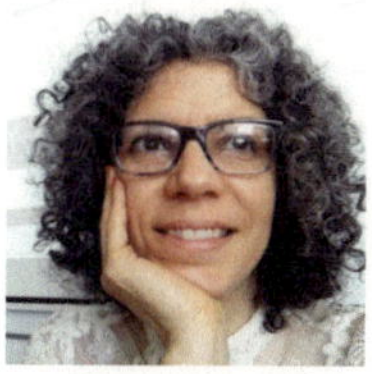

Aida Isabel Tavares holds a Ph.D. in Economic Analysis from the Autonomous University of Barcelona, Spain, and a Ph.D. in Management Science Applied to Decision Making from the University of Coimbra, Portugal. She has published several journal papers on applied health economics and two books, one on public economics and one on the obesity epidemic and the environment in Latin America. Dr. Tavares is also a book editor. Her research areas include health economics and policy, health systems, socio-economic determinants of health, regulation in health markets, and economic evaluation. She teaches courses on microeconomics, public economics, and health economics at different universities. Currently, she is a researcher at the Centre of Studies and Research in Health, University of Coimbra. She is also an assistant professor at the Lisbon School of Economics and Management, University of Lisbon, Portugal.

Contents

Preface

Health insurance is the mechanism used to respond to uncertainty and the risk of the consequences of illness. Health systems, which aim to promote population health and prevent people from financial collapse, are the umbrella structures that accommodate health insurance in each country. The variety of health systems around the world is large and each has its own features. There are public and private health insurances, voluntary or compulsory, and those financed by taxes, social compulsory contributions, or direct payments.

Differences in health insurance are significant between low-middle- and high-income countries. These differences mainly arise from the differences in the ability to finance the health insurance system. While high-income countries are typically able to finance and fund the provision of health care, low-medium-income countries face difficulty. Another challenge for these countries is the provision of universal health coverage (UHC), which is the United Nations' Sustainability Development Goal Target 3.8. As such, several countries are redesigning their health systems and focusing on strengthening them to support the priority of providing UHC.

This book discusses the path to redesign and reform health systems to achieve UHC. It is argued that the health insurance system plays a role in the move toward UHC. This progress may be financed by a combination of taxes and social health insurance contributions, as described in Chapter 1, "Toward Universal Health Coverage: The Role of Health Insurance System". The collected funds from these two sources are to be used in providing a basket of basic health care to satisfy population needs. Chapter 2, "The Advantage of Single-Payer National Insurance", also examines the problem of funding UHC in low-medium-income countries. It discusses different funding alternatives and describes the advantages of a single-payer national health insurance system, which is well-suited for those countries.

In low-medium-income countries, providing UHC under a health insurance system may be problematic because of the significant share of people who have very low incomes or work in the informal sector. Chapter 3, "Health Insurance for Economically Disadvantaged People in LMICs: What are the Best Options?", discusses the inequities emerging in these cases. This chapter proposes some measures to respond to this problem related to large informal sectors and a large share of poor people in the economy and society. Chapter 4, "National Health Insurance, the Informal Sector, and Elements of a New Social Contract in the 2019 UHC Act of the Philippines", presents the example of the Philippines and analyzes the different elements of the social contract for this country. Some of these elements may enhance or break down relationships in informal sector health insurance so that greater health security may be provided within the social contract context. Another area of concern within health systems is the allocation of funds and purchasing of services. Chapter 5, "An Assessment of the Effect National Health Insurance Scheme Capitation Payment to the Healthcare Facilities in Yobe State", presents a case study from Nigeria, the conclusions of which point to the benefits of the capitation payment mechanism. These benefits will increase competition among providers, reduce out-of-pocket payments, and guarantee the quality of services.

In high-income countries, the problems arising from providing UHC are different from those faced by low-middle-income countries. Chapter 6, "Complementary Health Insurance in Slovenia", presents the case for Slovenia. This country provides UHC financed by a compulsory contribution and a complementary health insurance scheme. The chapter examines the advantages and disadvantages of this special dual financing system. Chapter 7, "Voluntary Private Health Insurance Demand by Older People in a National Health Service, the Case of Portugal", presents the example of Portugal, which has a national health service financed by taxes and provides a UHC. The system faces some difficulties in ensuring the provision of UHC, and private voluntary health insurance is often a possible alternative. However, this alternative is quite limited to seniors. The chapter analyzes the main determinants for Portuguese seniors to buy private voluntary health insurance. Chapter 8, "Health Insurance in the United States: Failure of Private and Multi-Payer Financing", outlines the history of health insurance in the United States since the 1930s. It concludes that the not-for-profit and public single-payer Medicare for All can provide comprehensive coverage based on health care as a human right at affordable costs. Chapter 9, "Value-Based Contracting in Health Care", returns to the topic of concern within health systems about the allocation of funds and purchasing of services in the United States and other high-income countries. The issue examined in this chapter is the risk sharing between providers and payers using value-based contracting. These types of contracts ought to account for aspects such as prices, risk sharing, and outcome evaluation. Finally, Chapter 10, "Socio-Economic Considerations of Universal Health Coverage: Focus on the Concept of Health Care Value and Medical Treatment Price", examines the relationship between the progress of UHC and the socioeconomic factors promoting the sustainable development of health insurance systems. Based on this discussion, the chapter sets out the case of Japanese private clinical practices along with the consideration of the relationship between value and price, which is key to the future development of medical insurance systems.

Aida Isabel Tavares
ISEG, UL - Lisbon School of Economics and Management,
University of Lisbon,
Lisbon, Portugal

CEISUC - Centre for Health Studies and Research,
University of Coimbra,
Coimbra, Portugal

Section 1

Universal Health Coverage

Chapter 1

Toward Universal Health Coverage: The Role of Health Insurance System

Diriba Feyisa

Abstract

Health insurance is one of the instruments to achieve universal health coverage, which is not only the major goal for health reform in many countries but also the priority objective of World Health Organization. It provides financial security against healthcare costs and lessens the risk of incurring medical debt. There is an increasing understanding that poverty is exacerbated by ill health. Developing nations have recently increased the usage of various health insurance schemes to improve access to healthcare for low-income households to stop the negative downward circle of poverty and illness. These models help all countries regardless of income level can set out on the path to universal health coverage through a mix of different prepayment and risk-pooling mechanisms, tax-funding, and social health insurance. Right policies are necessary to achieve UHC. Concentrating on providing strong coverage for a clearly defined basket of services is well preferable to shallow coverage for every service with a high patient cost-sharing ratio. Health insurance system must be designed from the outset to be financially sustainable, which includes looking into ways to increase revenue sources and giving priority to the efficient use of resources.

Keywords: universal health coverage, health insurance system, healthcare financing, financial protection, out-of-pocket expenditure, access to healthcare

1. Introduction

Health is essential for leading a fruitful social and economic life [1]. Due to their direct impact on their ability to work, individuals' well-being is crucial for ensuring the welfare of the household as a whole, especially that of children [1]. Good health is the desired state for the wellness of human beings and to prolong economic, social, and political development pursuing a healthy society and global fastening. Healthcare access affects an individual's entire health condition, such as physical, mental, and social, as well as the overall quality of life [2].

According to the World Health Organization (WHO), access to healthcare services is a fundamental human right for every individual, and it is the responsibility of the government to make sure that these services are acceptable and readily available at all times [3]. Accessibility to healthcare services has various aspects that are influenced by service availability, the quality of patient care provided at health facilities, geographical connectivity, and economical mobility [3].

With significant regional diversity, there are combinations of health financing system consisting of public (tax-based systems, health insurance funds, and external funds) and private (mostly in the form of out-of-pocket payments) for financing healthcare worldwide. Prepayment model health financing systems are crucial for financial risk protection (FRP), which guarantees that people access healthcare without experiencing economic difficulties and are used by most high-income and middle-income nations. However, in low-income nations, these models are frequently inadequate and hence, many are excessively reliant on out-of-pocket payments, which put households at an elevated risk of financial difficulty and inequities in health outcomes [4, 5]. One hundred and fifty million individuals worldwide experience financial hardship due to the cost of healthcare services [6]. About 400 million individuals lack access to healthcare, and 8 million people lost their life due to preventable diseases, resulting in a loss of 6 trillion USD in economic productivity in low- and middle-income countries (LMICs) [6]. The sustainable development goals (SDGs) were adopted by world leaders in 2015, and these leaders strived toward achieving universal health coverage, which includes financial safeguards and access to inexpensive, high-quality critical medications [6].

The World Health Organization defines universal health coverage as the provision of preventive, curative, and rehabilitative health services without causing financial hardship when getting these services [7]. This process is challenging as it requires identifying the crucial elements that improve or degrade coverage, services, and reducing inequalities due to the abundance of players and the complexities of interactions that affect health coverage [8]. Therefore, to achieve the aims of UHC, strategies should be defined, formulated, and entrenched in various aspects of health financing policy environment. In this sense, the core of UHC is financial security, and enhancing safety net is a major goal of health financing policy. The framework, actions of key parties, and level of health outcomes are all defined by the type of healthcare financing used.

As a result, the finance model for healthcare is intimately and inextricably related to the delivery of health services, and it also serves to establish the upper limits of the system's capacity to meet the overarching objective of accelerating national economic growth [9]. Healthcare financing includes not just how to raise the necessary funds to meet a country's healthcare demands, but also how to assure fairness, affordability and accessibility of healthcare services, and financial risk mitigation. How health systems are financed largely determines whether people can obtain needed healthcare and whether they suffer financial hardship at the instance of obtaining care [10, 11].

2. Health financing and insurance system

The WHO created a framework for health financing that emphasizes the need for financing strategies to be assimilated into national health policies and service delivery plans [12]. Healthcare financing in LMICs and people's access to vital quality healthcare are dependent on OOPs, despite ongoing worldwide consensus over the need to enhance national health financing systems to build sustainable and all-encompassing policies. These obstacles to access are a major cause of preventable mortality [13].

To preserve and improve human wellbeing, health systems highly depend on health financing. Healthcare financing is the function of health system involved with the mobilization, accumulation, and funding to meet the health demands of the people, collectively and individually, in the health system [9]. Health insurance remains an imperative policy strategy for improving health outcomes at this crucial time, when many countries are pursuing the third sustainable development goal (SDG) of safeguarding healthy lives and promoting well-being for all at all ages [7, 14]. As a result, health insurance ensures that no one has to choose between getting medical care and going without for the sake of a lack of money [15, 16]. The World Bank has stated that several nations' sustainable development goals (SDGs) consider health insurance as a crucial component [17].

To guarantee that everyone has access to quality healthcare; the goal of health finance is to make funds accessible and to set the appropriate economic incentives for providers [11]. The health financing system frequently focuses on three interconnected essential features. The first is revenue collection: mobilizing sufficient resources from internal and external sources (such as prepayment schemes, government taxes, OOP payments, and donor funds). The second feature is risk pooling: the concentration and equitable distribution of prepaid economic resources to provide FRP across all beneficiaries, and pooled funds that can be derived from tax and donor funds. The third is fund allocation: allocating funding to health service providers will ensure that the public has access to adequate and effective services.

General tax income, social insurance, voluntary insurance, charity donations, and individual out-of-pocket costs are the five ways that health expenses are financed. To really achieve the intended advantages, countries' health benefit packages (HBPs) must be structured around the three essential components of the health funding system. Coordination between various funding sources is essential for attaining UHC given nations' health finance structures are typically combinations of public (tax-based, health insurance funds, and outside help) and private mechanisms (OOP) [7, 18].

The payment for healthcare at the time-of-service use is reduced and healthcare financing provides universal coverage of publicly supported essential health services. Additionally, by providing cross-subsidies from the wealthy to the poor and from the well-off to the ill, universal health funding would improve equity. Health financing and insurance reforms are being pushed in the favor of prepaid sources using general taxes, health insurance, or a combination of measures. However, development varies among nations, with public financing predominating in high-income nations and private expenditure being prevalent in LMICs [19].

Most nations are dedicated to building a strong health insurance system to achieve universal coverage. However, there is ongoing discussion over the relative merits of various types of health insurance (**Table 1**) [20]. The United Kingdom, for example, has developed a tax-based national health system that covers every resident [21].

Social health insurance on the other hand relies on employees contributing a percentage of their salaries to a health insurance fund that is used to refund affiliates' health expenditures [20–22]. Social insurance programs are mandatory insurance systems that are contributed to by employers and employees. Germany has created an extensive system of health, pension, long-term care, and insurance schemes for its inhabitants, providing a minimal degree of financial security that is frequently used as a benchmark for social insurance systems and advances the aspects of preventive care, primary prevention, resource, and financing decisions [23].

Private health insurance mostly appeals to the wealthy portions of the population and provides health plans that cover a certain list of medical issues in exchange for a renewable premium [20, 24].

Type of health insurance	Financing sources	Finance management	Underlying values and principles
National health insurance	General taxes	Public sector	Equity: equal access to health services for everyone
Social health insurance	Payroll taxes from employers and employees	Social security agency, national health fund, sickness funds	Solidarity: equal access to health services to all members of insurance fund
Private voluntary health insurance	Premium payments from individuals or employers/ employees	Commercial insurance company, for-profit or nonprofit organization	Principle of equivalence: health service provision with respect to ability to pay
Community health insurance	Premium payments from individuals or communities	Community or association	Constitute both part component of solidarity and principle of equivalence

Source: Authors' own construct following various literature reviews.

Table 1.
Major types of health insurance and health financing mechanism.

Organizations and/or employees may choose to obtain insurance from private companies voluntarily to reduce the possibility of monetary losses brought on by disease or the price of healthcare. Large portions of society in several nations have their health needs covered through voluntary insurance programs rather than social insurance programs. For instance, around two-thirds of the active population in the United States is covered by voluntary insurance.

Community-based health schemes are widespread in low- and middle-income nations and are frequently intended to help the underprivileged. In many nations, these programs are also utilized to raise additional funds to maintain disjointed health systems or diverse funding systems [20, 25].

Out-of-pocket funding for public health projects might not produce the best results. First, by eliminating the very obstacles to engagement that out-of-pocket costs offer, numerous healthcare businesses aim to boost disease management and promote health initiatives. Second, paying for healthcare out of pocket reveals what people are prepared to pay for a service and the amount they consume at that cost.

3. Universal health coverage

The 2030 Agenda for Sustainable Development was endorsed by the UN General Assembly in 2015 [26]. The 2030 Agenda emphasizes the significance of strengthening comprehensive and coherent methods to ensure that "no one is left behind" in obtaining universal health coverage (UHC). The agenda includes 17 sustainable development goals (SDGs) that must be accomplished [26].

Universal health coverage (UHC) articulates that everyone should have access to high-quality medical care that meets their requirements without experiencing economic difficulties. It asserts that a wide range of essential services is provided to the public in a way that is well connected with other social goals [17, 27].

Universal health coverage (UHC) as devoted to by the United Nations affiliate in the SDGs, can contribute to health equity if it is appropriately premeditated and realized [28, 29]. To achieve the overarching goal of good health and wellbeing for all people as well as other important healthcare targets in the SDGs, such as mortality reduction and the prevention of premature mortality from noncommunicable diseases. It is imperative that the two unmistakable goals of UHC; achieving equitable access to high-quality essential healthcare services and ensuring social financial risk protection be met [12].

WHO Report of 2019 called for all health systems to move toward universal coverage, defined as "access to adequate healthcare for all at an affordable price" [28]. Everyone wants access to high-quality, reasonable healthcare. The goal of UHC is to ensure that everyone has access to the medical services they require without facing financial hardship. Universal health coverage (UHC) seeks to improve health and community development, prevent disease from pushing people below the poverty line, and provide people the chance to live longer, healthier lives [15, 29, 30].

The objectives of UHC are to make sure that everyone has access to high-quality healthcare, to protect everyone from risks to the public's health, and to prevent

Target groups	**All people, including the poorest and most vulnerable**
Scope	Full range of essential health services, including prevention, treatment, hospital care, and pain control.
Accessibility	Costs are shared among the entire population through prepayment and risk-pooling, rather than shouldered by the sick. Physical accessibility, financial affordability, and social and cultural acceptability
Key aspects of the right to health	The right to health contains entitlements health services, goods, and facilities that must be provided to all without any discrimination. All services, goods, and facilities must be available, accessible, acceptable, and of good quality
Countries requirement	Pursuing policy reform political leadership and a clear strategic vision
Core Tenets	Prioritize the poorest, increase reliance on public funding, reduce, if not eliminate, out-of-pocket spending, and develop the health system
Approach	There is no one-size-fits-all approach. Countries are taking different pathways: strategies will depend on local circumstances and national dialogue.
A framework for action	Financing (more and better spending and effective financial protection), services (people-centered services, quality, and multisectoral action), equity (targeting the poor and marginalized and leaving no one behind), preparedness (strengthening health security) and governance (political and institutional foundations for the UHC agenda)
Impact	Improved health status, improved household financial wellbeing, increased responsiveness, and better health security
Challenges	Poverty

Sources: Authors' own construct following various literature reviews.

Table 2.
Summary of universal health coverage.

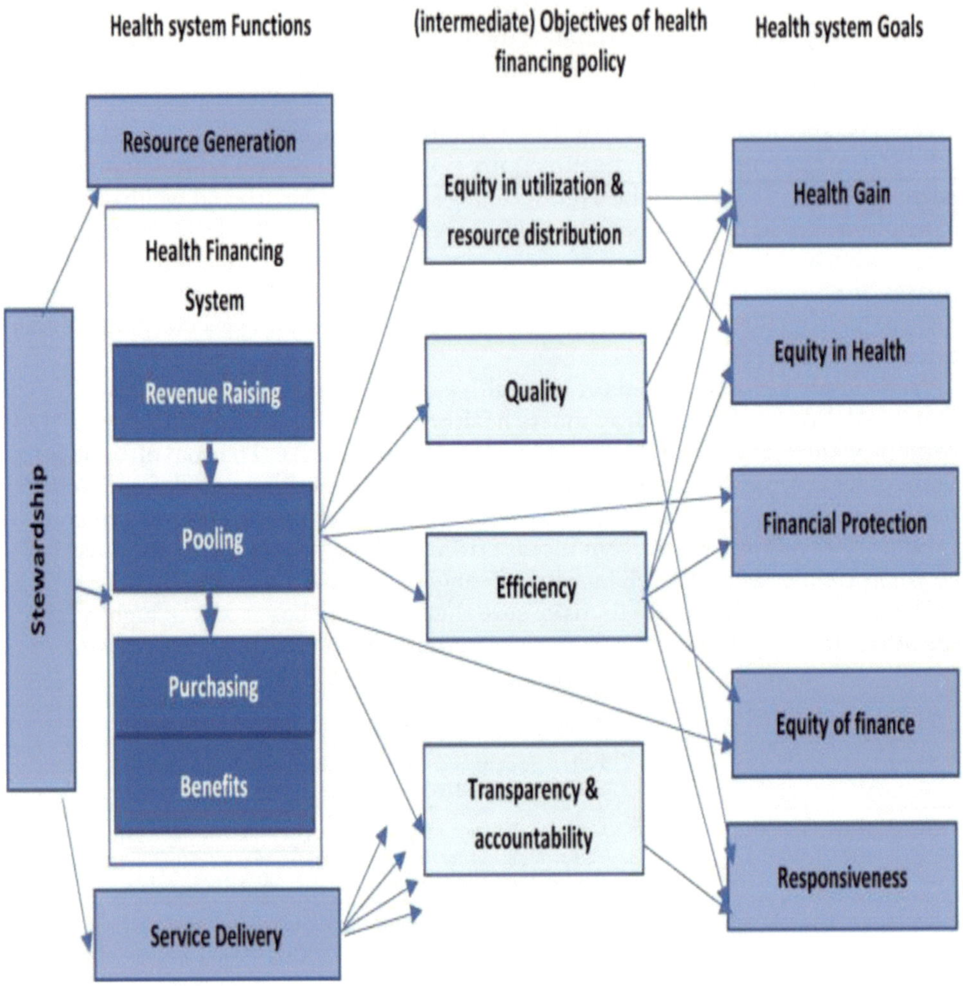

Figure 1.
Relationship among health system functions, healthcare financing policy, and universal health coverage as health system goal. Source: Kutzin, Joseph. Health financing for universal coverage and health system performance: concepts and implications for policy. Bulletin of the World Health Organization 2013;91:602-611.

everyone from falling into poverty because of illness, whether from out-of-pocket medical expenses or from lost income when a family member becomes ill. To reduce extreme poverty by 2030 and increase shared prosperity in lower- and medium-income countries (LMICs), where the majority of the world's poor reside, it will be crucial to provide universal access with quality and without financial obstacles (**Table 2**) [16, 31, 32].

Universal health coverage ranges of comprehensive services, including prevention, promotion, treatment, rehabilitation, and palliative care would progressively expand to reduce the unmet health needs, as no or few countries can afford to instantly finance a full set of services to all people [11, 12, 33]. UHC encompasses different health system components, including service delivery, financing policy, information system, infrastructure, health workforce, drug supply management, and governance (**Figure 1**) [11].

The road to UHC is not easy; each nation already has some systems in place, and in order to progress to UHC, each nation must strengthen those systems [11, 33]. Nevertheless, each nation must make progress in at least three different areas in order to meet the UHC objective: the first is the percentage of persons covered by pooled funds, the second is the range of accessible, and the third is cost-sharing from aggregated funds (**Figure 2**) [33].

Government ought to make important policy decisions as they proceed along these dimensions in order to improve effectiveness, be fair, and address other issues [10]. These decisions entail balancing how much of the population is addressed, the scope and types of care provided, and the cost covered by the aggregated money to achieve complete coverage in each dimension. Coverage along all three dimensions is achieved through risk pooling, health insurance, and/or government-financed provision of services (the blue cube within the UHC cube) [9].

Access to healthcare is used to measure whether people are receiving the services they need or not. It includes the physical availability and accessibility, economic affordability, and psycho-social acceptability of health services by the people. Accessible services also increase responsiveness, decrease health inequality, and improve health outcomes [31, 34]. According to WHO, about one-third of the world's population is without the access to medicines they need, mostly in Asia and Africa [4, 35].

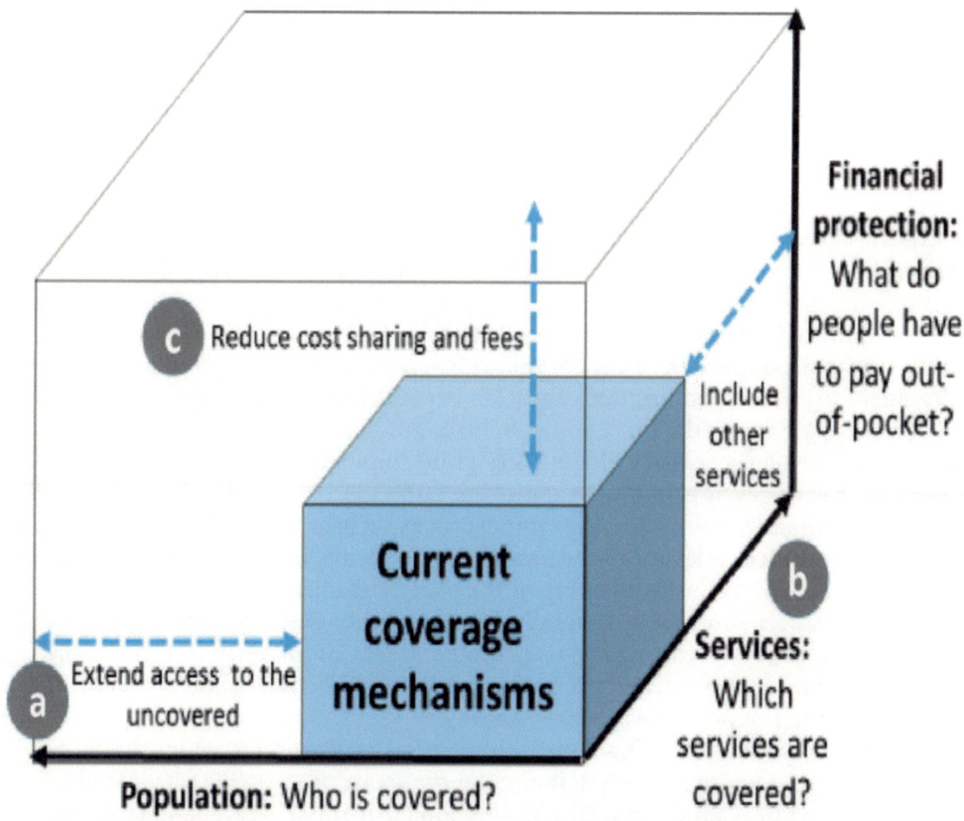

Figure 2.
Three dimensions to consider when moving toward universal coverage. Source: WHO (2010).

Globally, millions of people suffer and die due to lack of money to pay for healthcare while others suffer by paying more catastrophic payments. Accordingly, World Health Organization (WHO) recommends moving away from direct, out-of-pocket payments to using prepaid mechanisms to raise funds for health [12]. Every year, 100 million people are pushed into poverty because they have had to pay directly for their healthcare [19, 36, 37].

Today, a key element of national health strategy in numerous middle-income countries is achieving financial protection from risks related to family OOP expenditures on healthcare [38]. Financial risk protection represents the trade-off between funding essential requirements like schooling, nourishment, and housing on the one hand and paying for necessary health services on the other [4, 15]. A key goal of health insurance during era of universal health coverage is to reduce financial risks caused by high out-of-pocket health spending as the result of households' catastrophic healthcare payments that consume a large portion of their overall budget, eventually pushing them into poverty where they must take out loans or sell assets to pay for healthcare [4, 7, 37].

4. Health insurance system as a means of attaining universal health coverage

For many nations, health insurance is an integral component of the sustainable development goals (SDGs) [39]. In accordance to a 2017 World Health Organization (WHO) report, half of the planet's population cannot benefit from relevant health services, whereas about 100 million people per year are forced into chronic poverty as a consequence of medical expenses. Additionally, 800 million individuals spend roughly 10% of their family income on healthcare [7].

Fifty-eight (58) WHO World Health Assembly member nations resolved to expand their health-financing systems by increasing the role of prepayment for medical services while reducing direct payments, which were considered among the obstacles to accessing medical services [30]. Among the prepayment schemes, community-based health insurance (CBHI) is one that pools risks across different population groups so that the financial burden of catastrophic illnesses is significantly reduced for the individual [40]. CBHI reduces out-of-pocket expenditure and improves cost recovery, and it appears to be the most appropriate insurance model for informal sectors [40–42]. Balancing these three dimensions while emphasizing the quality and equity of the health services, is essential to achieving UHC [33].

UHC is, arguably, one of the most important aspects of equitable and fair access to healthcare services relevant to the needs of individuals. UHC program adoption has been reliant on a robust leadership of the party, detailing a variety of specific legislative, financial, and social tools all packed together that make the intervention successful and relevant from a long-term system integration viewpoint. Acquiring finances, pooling resources, and procuring services and benefit plans are some of the tasks involved in financing healthcare [43, 44].

However, achieving UHC is a journey of gradual realization in which everyone must advance on a variety of levels, including the scope of available services like medications, medical supplies, health professionals, infrastructure, and information as well as the percentage of covered cost and individuals [45, 46]. Therefore, to make progress, many stakeholders must be committed to working together and have the capacity to recognize and overcome hurdles. Health financing restructuring is vital and should be aimed at providing everyone with access to healthcare, offering financial protection, enhancing health outcomes, lowering the financial risks associated with illness, and boosting equity financing to overcome the current financial constraints to receiving medical care [12].

5. Policy implications

The United Nations sustainable development goals (specifically goal 3) and WHO's universal health coverage agenda, which is central to better health and well-being for all, delivering gains across 2030 sustainable development agenda that pledges to leave no one behind and realize improvement in health outcome, necessitates substantial changes in how each country finance both public health and the larger health system [17].

Ensuring that individuals are protected from the financial effects of illness, paying for healthcare as well as promoting the best use of available resources is the primary role of health insurance in meeting UHC goals. This is especially difficult given that both emerging and developed nations must increase healthcare services coverage to people that are not originally insured in order to attain these goals [7, 33].

As out-of-pocket payments are decreased; government agencies, insurer institutions, and private foundations are pressed to raise the resources dedicated to healthcare systems due to increment of insured individuals and expansion of health services coverage. The WHO has suggested a number of measures with the goals of boosting income, reducing obstacles, and improving efficiency to relieve this financial burden [33].

Boost the effectiveness of collecting money through strengthening revenue collection infrastructure and movement away from black and grey markets to a more stable environment where tax avoidance is minimized. This will boost the amount of money that government have at their disposal to finance population health.

For many reasons, UHC means the distinction between providing finance and privation of health services. It has been demonstrated that nations with expanded healthcare coverage have improved health indices and stronger overall socio-economic development. Since most of the voters demand access to inexpensive and high-quality health services, supporting a UHC agenda can result in significant electoral dividends for political leaders.

It is simple to forget that progress toward universal health coverage (UHC), is a political task that entails negotiations among different priority groups in society over the distribution of health benefits and resources to be consumed to gain such benefits as there are several complicated technical issues encountered on the way. Generally, moving toward achieving UHC offers health, economic, and political benefits [27, 47].

6. Conclusions

In conclusion, universal health coverage in terms of healthcare insurance function is physical and financial access to essential healthcare which are of good quality for all persons in the community. This implies protection against catastrophic expenditure on healthcare services are needed, services of good quality will be geographically accessible, and the costs of health services will not hinder people from using them or will not impoverish their families.

Effective healthcare finance solutions are essential, yet they are still difficult to implement sustainable health services. Realization of UHC is supported by appropriate health funding solutions that protect against financial risk.

Achieving effective and equitable UHC has a strong potential to improve and extend people's lives, reduce inequality, and potentially lead to economic growth. Failing to do just that may lead to deteriorating population health outcomes. UHC is more crucial than ever considering the unusual advent of the coronavirus disease 2019 (COVID-19) pandemic. Healthcare access and quality remain a challenge worldwide and efforts ought to make improve these issues through UHC are pivotal.

Conflict of interest

The author declares no conflict of interest.

Abbreviations

CBHI	community-based health insurance
FRP	financial risk protection
HBP	health benefit package
LMICs	low and middle-income countries
OOPs	out of pockets
UHC	universal health coverage
SDG	sustainable development goals
SHI	social health insurance
WHO	World Health Organization

Author details

Diriba Feyisa
Department of Medicine, College of Health Sciences, Salale University, Fiche, Ethiopia

*Address all correspondence to: diremask@gmail.com

References

[1] Asenso-Okyere K, Chiang C, Thangata P. Health interaction with farm labor productivity. 2011

[2] Peters DH, Garg A, Bloom G, Walker DG, Brieger WR, Hafizur Rahman M. Poverty and access to health care in developing countries. Annals of the New York Academy of Sciences. 2008;**1136**:161-171. DOI: 10.1196/annals.1425.011

[3] Allegheny County Health Department. Health equity brief access to health care in allegheny county why is access to health care important? 2018. Available from: https://www.alleghenycounty.us/uploadedFiles/Allegheny_Home/Health_Department/Resources/Data_and_Reporting/Chronic_Disease_Epidemiology/HEB-ACCESS.pdf

[4] Verguet S et al. Health gains and financial risk protection afforded by public financing of selected interventions in ethiopia: An extended cost-effectiveness analysis. The Lancet Global Health. 2015;**3**(5):e288-e296. DOI: 10.1016/S2214-109X(14)70346-8

[5] World Health Organization. Primary health care on the road to universal health coverage: 2019 global monitoring report: Executive summary. World Health Organization; 2019. Available from: https://www.who.int/publications/i/item/9789240029040%0Ahttps://www.who.int/docs/default-source/documents/2019-uhc-report.pdf

[6] Zegeye B et al. Breaking barriers to healthcare access: A multilevel analysis of individual- and community-level factors affecting women's access to healthcare services in Benin. International Journal of Environmental Research and Public Health. 2021;**18**(2):1-15. DOI: 10.3390/ijerph18020750

[7] World Health Organization (WHO). Tracking Universal Health Coverage: 2017 Global Monitoring Report. 2017. DOI: 10.1596/978-92-4-151355-5

[8] World Health Organization (WHO). The World Health Report 2006: Working together for health. Education for Health: Change in Learning and Practice. 2006;**19**(3):385-387. DOI: 10.1080/13576280600937911

[9] Riman HB, Akpan ES. Healthcare financing and health outcomes in Nigeria: A state level study using multivariate analysis. International Journal of Humanities and Social Science. 2012;**2**(15):296-309

[10] Carrin G, Evans D, Xu K. Designing health financing policy towards universal coverage. Bulletin World Health Organization. 2007;**85**(9):652

[11] Carrin G, Mathauer I, Xu K, Evans DB. Universal coverage of health services: Tailoring its implementation. Bulletin of the World Health Organization. 2008;**86**(11):857-863. DOI: 10.2471/BLT.07.049387

[12] Kutzin J. Health financing for universal coverage and health system performance: Concepts and implications for policy. Bulletin of the World Health Organization. 2013;**91**(8):602-611. DOI: 10.2471/BLT.12.113985

[13] Beattie A, Yates R, Noble DJ. Accelerating progress towards universal health coverage in Asia and Pacific: Improving the future for women and children. BMJ Global Health.

2016;**1**(Supp 2):I12-I18. DOI: 10.1136/bmjgh-2016-000190

[14] Al-Hanawi MK, Mwale ML, Kamninga TM. The effects of health insurance on health-seeking behaviour: Evidence from the Kingdom of Saudi Arabia. Risk Management and Healthcare Policy. 2020;**13**:595-607. DOI: 10.2147/RMHP.S257381

[15] Saksena P, Hsu J, Evans DB. Financial risk protection and universal health coverage: Evidence and measurement challenges. PLoS Medicine. 2014;**11**:595

[16] McIntyre D, Ranson MK, Aulakh BK, Honda A. Promoting universal financial protection: Evidence from seven low- and middle-income countries on factors facilitating or hindering progress. Health Research Policy System. 2013;**11**(1):1

[17] UNDP. Universal health coverage for sustainable development. 2019

[18] Reich MR et al. Moving towards universal health coverage: Lessons from 11 country studies. Lancet. 2016;**387**(10020):811-816. DOI: 10.1016/S0140-6736(15)60002-2

[19] World Health Organization (WHO). Global Spending on Health: A World in Transition 2019. Glob. Rep. 2019. Available from: https://www.who.int/health_financing/documents/health-expenditure-report-2019/en/

[20] OXFAM. Universal health coverage: Why health insurance schemes are leaving the poor behind. In: OXFAM Brief. Pap. Vol. 176. 2013. p. 36

[21] Wagstaff. Social health insurance enrollement. Vol. 1131. 2008. pp. 1127-1131. DOI: 10.1002/hec

[22] Witter S, Garshong B. Something old or something new? Social health insurance in Ghana. BMC International and Health Human Rights. 2009;**9**(1):1186

[23] World Health Organization. Self-assessment tool for the evaluation of essential public health operations in the WHO European Region. In: Copenhagen World Heal. Organ. Reg. Off. Eur. 2015

[24] Sekhri N, Savedoff W. Private health insurance: Implications for developing countries. Bulletin of the World Health Organization. 2005;**83**(2):127

[25] Alexander EB, Preker S, Liu X, Edit V. Public ends, private means: Strategic purchasing of health services. 2007

[26] United Nations. Transforming our world: The 2030 agenda for sustainable development. In: Arsen. Res. Glob. Sustain. - Proc. 6th Int. Congr. Arsen. Environ; New York, United Nations; 2016. pp. 12-14

[27] World Health Organization. Arguing for universal health coverage. 2013

[28] Garrett L, Chowdhury AMR, Pablos-Méndez A. All for universal health coverage. Lancet. 2009;**374**(9697):1294-1299. DOI: 10.1016/S0140-6736(09)61503-8

[29] World Health Organization and The World Bank. Global Monitoring Report on Financial Protection in Health 2019 Advance Copy [Online]. 2020. Available from: https://www.who.int/healthinfo/universal_health_coverage/report/fp_gmr_2019.pdf?ua=1

[30] Lozano R et al. Measuring universal health coverage based on an index of effective coverage of health services in 204 countries and territories, 1990-2019: A systematic analysis for the Global Burden of Disease Study 2019. Lancet.

2020;**396**(10258):1250-1284. DOI: 10.1016/S0140-6736(20)30750-9

[31] Tangcharoensathien V, Mills A, Palu T. Accelerating health equity: The key role of universal health coverage in the sustainable development goals. BMC Medicine. 2015;**13**(1):1-5. DOI: 10.1186/s12916-015-0342-3

[32] Akiko Maeda S, Araujo E, Harris J. Universal health coverage for inclusive and sustainable development: A synthesis of 11 country case studies. 2014. DOI: 10.1596/978-1-4648-0408-3

[33] World Health Organization (WHO). Making fair choices on the path to universal health coverage

[34] Kirton J, Kickbusch I. Health A Political Choice. Glob. Gouv. Progr. [Online]. 2019. pp. 1-132. Available from: http://edition.pagesuite.com/html5/reader/production/default.aspx?pubname=&edid=1b1471a7-7575-4371-9969-9e93f7dd4aa8

[35] Satti SA, Mohamed-Omer SF, Hajabubker MA. Pattern and determinants of use of traditional treatments in children attending Gaafar Ibnauf Children's Hospital, Sudan. Sudan Journal of Paediatric. 2016;**16**:45-50. Available from: http://www.ncbi.nlm.nih.gov/pubmed/28096558%0Ahttp://www.pubmedcentral.nih.gov/articlerender.fcgi?artid=PMC5237834

[36] N. Experiments. Editorial: Identification of treatment effects. Vol. 1131. 2008. pp. 1127-1131. DOI: 10.1002/hec

[37] Xu K, Evans DB, Kawabata K, Zeramdini R, Klavus J, Murray CJL. Household catastrophic health expenditure: A multicountry analysis. Lancet. 2003;**362**(9378):111-117. DOI: 10.1016/S0140-6736(03)13861-5

[38] Nundoochan A, Thorabally Y, Monohur S, Hsu J. Impact of out of pocket payments on financial risk protection indicators in a setting with no user fees: The case of Mauritius. International Journal for Equity in Health. 2019;**18**(1):1-11. DOI: 10.1186/s12939-019-0959-5

[39] Morton S, Pencheon D, Squires N. Sustainable development goals (SDGs), and their implementation. British Medical Bulletin. 2017;**124**(1):81-90. DOI: 10.1093/bmb/ldx031

[40] Tesfaye G. The Impact of Community Based Health Insurance in Health Service Utilization in Tigray: A Case of Kilte Awlaelo Woreda. Department of Economics, College of Business and Economics; 2014. p. 23

[41] Minyihun A, Gebregziabher MG, Gelaw YA. Willingness to pay for community-based health insurance and associated factors among rural households of Bugna District, Northeast Ethiopia. BMC Research Notes. 2019;**12**(1):1-7. DOI: 10.1186/s13104-019-4091-9

[42] Gidey MT, Gebretekle GB, Hogan ME, Fenta TG. Willingness to pay for social health insurance and its determinants among public servants in Mekelle City, Northern Ethiopia: A mixed methods study. Cost Effectiveness and Resources Allocation. 2019;**17**(1):1-11. DOI: 10.1186/s12962-019-0171-x

[43] Hallalo HA. Achieving universal health coverage through health financing reform: Ethiopian showcase. Health Economics and Outcome Research. 2018;**04**(01):1-5. DOI: 10.4172/2471-268x.1000148

[44] W. H. O. (WHO) UNICEF. Measuring progress on the pathway to universal. 2018

[45] Global Monitoring Report on Financial Protection in Health 2021. DOI: 10.1596/36723

[46] Okech TC, Lelegwe SL. Analysis of universal health coverage and equity on health care in Kenya. Global Journal of Health Science. 2015;**8**(7):218-227. DOI: 10.5539/gjhs.v8n7p218

[47] Moreno-Serra R, Smith PC. Does progress towards universal health coverage improve population health? Lancet. 2012;**380**(9845):917-923. DOI: 10.1016/S0140-6736(12)61039-3

Section 2

Health Insurance in Low-Medium Income Countries

Chapter 2

The Advantage of Single-Payer National Insurance

Hasbullah Thabrany and Mutia Sayekti

Abstract

The world leaders have committed to achieve universal health coverage as set on the goal of 3.8 of the SDGs by 2030. Only public financing could achieve UHC for everyone in a country. There are three sources of public financing, i.e., tax-funded or national health service system, social health insurance applied national or national health insurance scheme, and a combination of the two. Low- and middle-income countries are often easier to start with social health insurance schemes with multiple and single schemes. The option of a single-payer National Health Insurance scheme has a lot of advantages in terms of effectiveness, efficiencies, and equitable health financing for all people in a country. This chapter explains the rationales of health financing and options of public financing with various levels of the impacts on the people in particular and the country. A single-payer system facilitates easy understanding and ensures equitable access with the same benefits for everybody. A single-payer system also potentially has monopsony powers to ensure cost-effective health care. Expenditures data demonstrate relatively lower among single-payer systems with the relatively the similar health outcomes.

Keywords: health financing, health insurance, equitable health financing, single-payer national health insurance, universal health coverage

1. Introduction

Leaders of the world have committed to achieve universal health coverage (UHC) goal number 3.8 of the sustained development goals (SDGs) by 2030. This means that people of any country should have access to at least essential health services regardless of their income or social groups within a country. Two indicators are used in monitoring the UHC covering indicator 3.81 of service coverage and indicator 3.8.2 of catastrophic health spending [1, 2]. Service coverage ensures that everyone should have essential health services when she/he needs them and catastrophic health spending ensures that no one goes bankrupt when paying for health care to meet his/her need. Recent monitoring by three global organizations, the World Health Organization, the World Bank, and the OECD have demonstrated the progress of the incidence of catastrophic health spending with two thresholds percentage of 10% and 25% of the total household incomes or expenditures [3]. Catastrophic health spending (CHS) is an important measure of out-of-pocket (OOP) expenditure by household members that should not exceed 10% of income [4]. Above that, the household may become impoverished. The indicator 3.8.2 is essential to protect people from being poor due to the consumption of health care when ill health or accident occurs.

Market mechanism in health care means that everyone must purchase health care out of his/her pocket and the health care providers set prices above the production costs to get profit and develop the business. Because of the uncertain needs for health care, ability to pay at the prices set by the sellers (health care providers) market mechanism tend to impoverish people. The WHO reported that 996 million people in the world (13.2%) spend more than 10% of their budget on OOP health care consumption [5]. Health economic literatures have long acknowledged that health care is not normal goods because of its unique characteristics. For the normal goods or services, market mechanism leads a fair competition and to adequate supplies the people could purchase, lower prices and higher quality of products. One of the requirements of perfectly competitive market is the information symmetry between the purchasers and the sellers.

There are three main distinct characteristics of health care needs that make fully competitive market mechanism of health care does not function well [6]. The first characteristic is *uncertainty* of health care needs in terms of time in the future, location, amount of money, and amount of health care consumed. Health care consumption may be affordable if the ill-health is mild, but it can be devastating to an individual's wealth or income if someone is suffering from severe illness such as heart attack, stroke, or cancer. In an insurance theory, an uncertain future event with large financial risks can be transferred to an insurer as in insurance mechanism by paying premium or contribution [7, 8]. The amount of premium is an average expected amount of money, which relatively small amount and affordable, to cover financial risks of an insured population. For example, in a simplified commercial health insurance scheme, an insurer may sell single benefit of renal transplant with the average cost of $100,000 and the probability of occurrence of renal failure that required renal transplant in that community is one per 10,000 population. The pure or net premium (no loading factor to cover administrative, marketing, and profits) will be $10 ($100,000 multiple with 1/10,000 probability). By paying $10 premium, a person will be insured to afford a renal transplant, once s/he suffers from a renal failure.

There are two main types of health insurance based on the mandatory or voluntary transfer of risks. The mandatory insurance scheme is called social health insurance, which is normally used in national health insurance (NHI), while the voluntary joining health insurance is called commercial health insurance. Another way of managing risk of uncertainty in health care is to cover all health care needs by the state budget like in the National Health Service (NHS) scheme in the United Kingdom [9].

Health insurance can be differentiated according to the financing function of the health system. There are systems mainly financed by taxes while others are mainly financed by social health insurance (SHI). Both income tax and SHI contribution are compulsory in the world. Both SHI and income tax are taken proportionally from income or salaries. To top up those mandatory contributions, in many countries, there are markets for private (voluntary) health insurance, except in few countries such as the United States where private health insurance is the main source of health care financing for working population. However, for the elderly population with high health risks, the US health care system uses mandatory of a kind of SHI (the Medicare Program) [9, 10].

The second distinct characteristic of health care is the very high *asymmetric information*. Information symmetry is the key to a fully competitive market mechanism that leads to lower prices and higher quality of products or services. The symmetry of information facilitates a buyer to choose a product or service to be purchased. When a buyer has a lack of information, she/he could ask the details of the product, the benefit of the product, and compare prices with other products or substitutions or bargain the seller for the price. The buyer of a normal product makes his/her decision to purchase or consume fully or partially according to his/her ability to pay or his/her "perceived needs" with no harm. In health care, this independent and fully informed choice does not happen. In a market mechanism, an ordinary patient is unable to get full information about his/her needs, choices of appropriate health care, the fair price, the benefit, and the adverse effect of a health care she/he will consume. But the doctor (independent or representing a health care provider) knows much more, and at the same time, the doctor is advocating the patient what to consume. This very high asymmetric information between the patient (the buyer) and the doctor (the seller) poses a threat of moral hazard, abuse, and fraudulence act due to financial/profitable interests of the seller. This information asymmetry is the main cause of market failure [10].

What about health insurance market? It has also high information asymmetry. At the individual level, an individual has very little knowledge about the probability of health care needs covered by a health insurance policy, its appropriate premium, and how good is the insurance policy paying health care providers. The main drawback of private or commercial health insurance schemes is how an individual (called a prospect) understands his or her health risks and how much of these risks can be transferred, method of risk calculation to set premium, and how the insurer underwrites the health risks. Therefore, private health insurance is normally sold as group insurance, either as the main health care protection or as a top-up coverage in the NHI or NHS scheme. In commercial health insurance, the purchasing mechanism for individuals follows the "take it or leave it" business model. Both commercial health insurance and health care do not meet the requirement of independent decision to purchase health care or health insurance. Since the nature of transaction of commercial insurance is voluntary and insurers are companies seeking profits, commercial health insurance schemes are always multipayers. Every business entity has a freedom to enter the health insurance market. A health system that depends heavily on commercial health insurance will not achieve effective (cover all people or UHC) and efficient health system (a relative low portion of GDP is spent for health). Designing, marketing, and managing commercial health insurance require multiple professional workers, and the economy of scale will not achieve efficient system. Competition in health insurance market pushes insurers to create unique and competitive plans (health insurance products) leading to only portions of people or groups of people that may purchase. This condition absolutely will not achieve the law of a large number of the main predictable events of insurance principle.

The third distinct characteristic of health care is the *externalities* of health care consumption or products. An externality occurs when a person consumes a good or a service and there are effects created on other people with are not expressed in the price. *Positive externality* occurs, for instance, if a tuberculosis patient consumes medication, people around him/her will benefit for not being contacted by TB. On the other hand, a *negative externality* may occur if someone regularly smokes cigarettes that risk his/her heart or lungs or cause cancer, and other people around him/her who inhale the smoke will be subject to a higher risk of tobacco-related diseases (TRDs). This externality poses unfairness of purchasing health care. It is not fair to pay for treatment of TRDs when someone has never smoked. Therefore, externality becomes the basis for public subsidy or public finance. Since it is difficult to identify who was causing negative impact of smoking, the application of sin tax [11] for health care is commonly practiced in many countries. Sin tax is a term used in some countries to signify that consumption of certain products such as tobacco or alcohol negatively affects health of the people. To reduce such negative externality of consumption of tobacco or alcohol, a financial disincentive called tax or excise is charged to the consumers. The term "earmarked tax" is used if a portion or whole of the sum of money collected from sin tax is dedicated by law to finance health services.

The combination of the three distinct characteristics of health care generates other unique health care needs called "patient ignorance, patient short-sighted, patient inability to pay, unfair health financing, and provider moral hazard or fraud." In addition, because unmet health care needs could result in severe disability or death, health care consumption is a human right. Therefore, combination of those unique characteristics of health care needs requires collective efforts and public funding. The goal of 3.8 of SDGs, UHC is the global commitment to meet health care needs for everyone. One of the key element of UHC is public financing using insurance mechanisms or tax-funded system.

2. Health insurance contract

Generally, many people think health insurance is commercial insurance, which is a rational and good instrument to overcome uncertainty of health care needs, especially in high-cost health care. Not many people understand social health insurance (SHI) schemes as a solution to financing health care for everyone. Some Muslim leaders and scholars (those who are preaching Islamic religion) mistakenly consider health insurance as not meeting Sharia requirements. Some of them understand health insurance as a trade of intangible products which violates the principle of Sharia, the Islamic law. In a narrow definition, a health insurance policy is a commercial transaction between one party to an institution called insurer of an intangible product or service which consider *gharar* in Islamic thought. However, current Muslim scholars agree to modify the meeting of mind of insurance contract as *hibah*, or donation for general benefit of all members of insurance. This school of thought then delivers an Islamic version of insurance mechanism called *takaful*, based on mutual help principle. In western countries, this mutual help is called a risk-sharing arrangement.

In wider definition of minimizing uncertainty, a publicly funded health care system such as the NHS can be considered providing health insurance for all people. When a country provides UHC using funding from general tax revenue, there is no uncertainty of health care needs at an individual level in the country applying NHS model. However, not all countries are able to establish and finance an NHS model. Many low and middle-income countries are looking for financing schemes that gradually meet the health care needs of all people in the country. One of the essential elements of the objectives of UHC is equity health financing, which means that financing for health care by individual is based on the ability of an individual to contribute (to pay), but the health care services consumed by the individual are based on his/her health care needs. This equitable financing can only be achieved by publicly funded system, based on tax-funded or social health insurance (SHI) mechanism. Once there is a pool-fund, the purchasing of health care for everyone should be managed effectively and efficiently.

Some country leaders may be trapped to rely on commercial health insurance (CHI) instead of SHI. Basically, both CHI and SHI share the characteristics of insurance contracts. The key difference between CHI and SHI is nature of entering into insurance contract. The CHI is voluntary transaction while the SHI is mandatory for individuals to enter into an insurance contract. Another key difference between CHI and SHI is the premium for CHI is based on the levels of health risks while the premium (often called "contribution") for SHI is based on a proportion of individual income or salary. The SHI can be implemented using multiple or single organizations. If the SHI scheme is administered by a single organization, a government agency, or a quasi-government organization, it is called a National Health Insurance (NHI) such as implemented in South Korea, Taiwan, the Philippines, and Indonesia. In many other countries, the SHI schemes are administered by various organizations such as implemented in Germany, French, and Japan.

An insurance contract stipulates right and obligation that bind each party. There are four distinct insurance contracts applicable to CHI and SHI: *conditional, unilateral, aleatory,* and *adhesion* [12, 13]. Both CHI and SHI schemes share at least three types of contracts. The main difference between CHI and SHI contract is the CHI use contract called *insurance policy* while the SHI utilizes regulation to mandate every individual in the country to join SHI. Both insurance policy (contract) and regulation of SHI provide rights and obligations of individuals and the insurers, insurance agencies, or administrators.

Due to the uncertain nature of health care needs, the obligation of an insurer (both CHI and SHI) is *conditional* upon the occurrence of an illness or accident generating health care needs. This conditional contract needs deep understanding of all people to implement an NHI scheme to comply with regular contributions, even if they are healthy and have never utilized the benefit for years. In Indonesia, at the beginning of the implementation of SHI, many people questioned, where their money goes (of contribution paid) for many years, despite they have never used any benefits. Many Islamic scholars question this conditional nature as not meeting the Islamic Sharia law creating challenges in countries with significant number of Muslim populations.

The 2nd characteristic of the insurance contract is *unilateral*. This unilateral contract is to compensate conditional contract that in favor of the insurer. Only insurer can be contested by policyholder if the insurer fails to meet its obligation. Policyholders could not be contested to the court for failure to pay contribution. It simply lapses the contract, and no benefit could be utilized by the policyholder.

The 3rd characteristic of insurance contract is *aleatory* meaning the asymmetry in rights and obligations of parties (insured and insurer). This aleatory contract legally allows unequal rights and obligations of the amount of money of insured and insurer. In CHI scheme, a policyholder may pay premium for only months (say $100 per month) then she/he suffers from heart attack and $100,000 for a bypass cardiac surgery, there is no obligation for the policyholder to make up the $99,800 difference. The insurer's right is only a two-month premium of $200 (which is the obligation of the insured). The insured right is $100,000 worth of surgical procedures, although the insured only pay $200. On the other hand, if the insured continuously receive premiums for 20 consecutive years of $100 per month (so total is 12 months x $ 100 x 20 years = $ 24,000) but she/he has never suffered from any illness—never claim (the trigger for the obligation of the insurer), the insurer has no obligation to return the $ 24,000 money the insured had paid the premium. A similar aleatory characteristic also applies in SHI scheme.

It is this contract that differs from the term of prepayment that is often used in some health care financing papers. The term "prepaid health care" was first used by Paul Ellwood in the USA for the Health Maintenance Organization (HMO) contract in 1973 just to get acceptance by the American Medical Association that opposed health insurance scheme at that time [14]. The term "prepayment" may be misleading to describe health care financing because of this aleatory contract. The term prepaid or prepayment as often used in mobile phone business is appropriate because the payer can consume phone service up to the amount paid in advance.

The last characteristic of insurance contract is called *adhesion*, in which one party is much weaker than the other. It is a type of information asymmetry where the prospect (a person who will purchase insurance) has no way to negotiate the price or the benefit. It is simply a "take it or leave it" transaction. Because of this contract nature, insurance businesses are heavily regulated to protect policyholders from unfair business practices by insurers. In SHI scheme detailed regulation is needed and oversight commission is in place to ensure that policyholders or members of SHI receive fair treatment.

3. Financing for UHC

Financing UHC using traditional health insurance concept of CHI poses significant problems. The double information asymmetry of health care need and health insurance contract create market failure to ensure everyone is covered to meet his/her health care needs. The unique characteristics of health care needs and the long-term externality of having healthy lives as the main requirement for individual economic productivity push all governments to ensure health services are available for everyone regardless of individual income or social status. The COVID-19 Pandemic has demonstrated how strong the health sector affected the World economy which declined by 3.4 percent in 2020 [15]. The COVID-19 pandemic emphasizes the importance of UHC as a set of the 3.8 Goal of SDGs. The UHC can only be achieved if there is sufficient public health financing.

There are three possible public financing for health that allow UHC with different efficiency levels. The first automatic covering all people is the tax funded or NHS model; the second one is the mature SHI model; and the third one is a combination of the two. Often SHI model is complemented with tax funded subsidies for the low-income people. The administration of funds of the SHI model varies widely across the countries with dominant SHI model. Currently, no country with CHI model could fully achieve UHC. There are differences in funding UHC based on health financing mechanisms as shown in the following **Table 1**.

The main problem of CHI is the voluntary nature of participation. People are shortsighted and health risks cannot be predicted by individual. Therefore, there is unlikely that an individual will purchase CHI or private health insurance coverage. But when someone suffers from a chronic condition, then that person will demand CHI creating adverse or anti selection. The insurer that aims for profit making certainly will undertake rigorous underwriting to ensure no adverse selection. The insurer may inherently design a benefit package, terms, and conditions for prospects to minimize adverse selection. Certainly, people suffering from a chronic condition elderly and those who have congenital health problems will not be able to purchase health insurance. In addition, because the premiums (prices) are set based on health risks of individuals or small groups, higher risks of individuals or small groups must

Element/Issue	CHI	SHI–NHI	NHS
Participation	Voluntary	Mandatory	Automatic
Ability to cover all population (UHC)	Almost impossible	Highly likely	Always
Inclusiveness	Almost impossible	Highly likely	Always
Benefit package	Vary widely, designed by the insurer	Relatively uniform for all people	Uniform for all
Nature of benefit package	Based on demand, Consideration of profit, mostly not comprehensive	Based on health care needs, mostly comprehensive	Subject to amount of state funds and health needs
Risk transfer / funding method	Risk-based premium	Income-based contribution, normal percentage of income	Income tax and other state taxes
Insurer	Private for-profit or not-for-profit	Private organization not for profit or government/ public entity	The government
Number of payers	Always multiple	Single or multiple	Always single there are regional payers in some cases
Legal basis	Various regulations on various aspects	Mostly by single regulation for all people or group of people	Constitution or state budget regulation
Administrative costs	High	Very low	Mix with state expenses
Adverse selection	Inherent, likely	Avoided	Avoided

Table 1.
Comparison between CHI, SHI, and NHS model.

pay higher premiums. This certainly excludes low-income people from having health insurance coverage. Commercial health insurance charge loading fees is significantly high, depending on the size of the group insured that can vary up to 34% of the total premiums paid [16]. Therefore, CHI model fails to achieve UHC.

Because of the market failure of CHI and health care market, the option to cover everyone is by public financing. Public financing is based on mandatory contribution and based on the proportion of income or wealth. There are only two funding mechanisms of publicly funded health care, which are the SHI model and the NHS model.

The SHI model could apply for certain group of employed population. For example, before the implementation of NHI in Indonesia, the civil servants were covered by Askes—the SHI scheme for government employees and the private employees were covered by another SHI scheme called Jamsostek. Another example is Thailand, private employees are covered under Social Security Scheme administered by the Ministry of Labor, and the informal sector is covered by a tax fund administered by the National Health Security Office Taiwan [17]. The Philippines, South Korea, and Indonesia used to have several SHI schemes before they were integrated into a single national SHI called NHI. The level of contribution for the NHI model is normally uniform, a portion of salary for all employees. In Indonesia, current contribution is 5% of monthly income, shared by employees (1%) and employers 4%. In Germany, with multiple sickness funds, current contribution levels at around 14.6%, shared 50: 50 by employers and employees [18].

The United Kingdom initiated the NHI model in 1911 and then started the NHS in 1948 administered by the state. The NHS model is normally funded by progressive income taxes, which often exceed 50% of monthly income for the high tier of income. Low and middle-income countries often have problems in collecting and enforcing high progressive income tax. The maximum level of income taxes in European Countries that implement NHS varies from 43% in Italy to 56.95% in Finland [19]. Certainly, many low- and middle-income countries (LMICs) could afford this model. But, still some LMICs such as Sri Lanka apply the NHS model even though the income tax level has been relatively low at 18%.

As an option to cover health care needs, many LMICs could start SHI model based on employment. The SHI was first introduced in Germany, called statutory health insurance, by Otto von Bismarck the chancellor of liberal party in 1883 [20]. However, at that time, Von Bismarck mandated contributions to pay income loss of a laborer who was suffering from serious sickness and unable to work for income. At that time most labor forces were based on daily paid work. Now, the SHI covers health care costs, which vary from limited hospitalization to comprehensive medical and family benefit. In Germany, since the SHI concept was introduced, there are multiple funds called sickness funds but in decreasing number [21]. In many countries, most SHI started to mandate large-size employers such as civil servants and private employers with more than 100 employees to contribute a portion of incomes to cover defined health care benefits. South Korea [22], Indonesia [7], Taiwan [23], and the Philippines [24], for example, started to mandate public and formal sector employees, years before mandating the informal sector to contribute to the single-payer NHI.

4. Single-payer National Health Insurance Scheme

In most LMICs where tax-funded system is not the option taken by the political leadership, SHI schemes can be a good choice to ensure equitable access to essential health care in LMICs. The SHI model can be gradually implemented for employed population for partial health benefits that the population can afford. Indonesia started SHI for civil servants in 1968 and then for private employees in 1993 and finally for everybody in 2014 [7]. China also introduced this social insurance model starting for employed groups. The challenges in implementing SHI for whole population are collecting contributions for the informal sector. The informal sector or non-waged earners do not have a regular monthly income. In LMICs, the proportion of non-waged earners is generally very high, more than 50%. Therefore, scaling up to cover the whole population to achieve UHC in LIMCs may take decades. One option is to subsidize the informal sector from the government budget, integrated to the NHI. When a country implementing SHI became a high-income country, normally the SHI model is continued to be implemented as happened in Germany, Korea, Japan, the Philippines, and Taiwan.

The choice of administrators of the SHI can be implemented by special SHI fund for special groups such as civil servants, private employees, teachers, farmers, etc. Multiple payer systems create possibility that some groups will have more coverage with higher contribution levels than others. Different SHI and different groups of population create oligo- or multi-payer systems that may provide problems in negotiating prices of health care from various providers. The Japan employer-based health insurance system creates a virtual single payer by forcing all SHI plans to purchase health care organized by Central Administrative Offices. Regardless of the plans, all

Japan's residents could go to the same health care providers. Implementing different SHI for different groups may create unequal benefits across different population groups and may not be acceptable in some countries. On the other hand, some small differences of contribution or preventive services like implemented in Japan are socially accepted [25]. Germany once had more than 5000 sickness funds; they now have less than 100 sickness funds. To ensure equity across different employment groups, Germany requires equalizing funds across different sickness funds [26]. South Korea once followed the German and Japan SHI model with multiple plans then in early 2000 integrated all SHI schemes into a single NHI model [14].

The politics, cultural values, social norms, and the national constitutions of countries play crucial roles in determining single- or multi-payer system of NHI. Indonesia also followed the Korean model, integrating SHI and social assistance schemes into a single NHI. The fight to establish a single NHI in Indonesia involved union strikes, extensive academic debates, and legal battle in the parliament and in the constitutional court [7]. Despite of the very high health expenditures, the USA has not achieved UHC. Only the elderly population is covered by the public fund of SHI model, called Medicare. The poor are covered by sharing of federal and state funds. The Obama Care is basically providing tax incentive for the informal sector to purchase CHI. Turkey integrates all SHI plans into a single NHI in 2008 by reforming the social security system [27].

5. Advantages of a single-payer NHI

In the last 30 years, four Asian countries started innovative health reform by establishment of a single-payer NHI. Taiwan started to implement the NHI in 1995, managed by the Bureau of the National Health Insurance of the Ministry of Health, providing comprehensive health care benefits [28]. Then, the Philippines followed in 1997 by establishing PhilHealth, the NHI Corporation attached to the Ministry of Health providing inpatient care only [29]. South Korea integrated more than 300 SHI plans into the NHI Service in 2000 providing comprehensive benefits with relatively high cost-sharing [30]. Indonesia followed enacting the national social security reform including the NHI in 2004 with comprehensive health care benefits, including preventive care. However, the political battles delayed the implementation of the NHI scheme (called JKN, *Jaminan Kesehatan Nasional)* in 2014 [7]. The single-payer NHI has several advantages as follows:

1. Meeting the Constitution mandate, which normally provides the right to health care for everyone. When the Constitution requires that every citizen has the right to health care, a single NHI could purchase health care from public and private health care providers, providing equitable access to meeting health care needs. The NHS model often limits access to public health care providers, while the single-payer NHI ensures the same access to everyone using any health care resources in the country.

2. The single-payer NHI has the biggest (monopsony) power to purchase health care from any health care providers licensed in the country [7, 31]. With this monopsony power, the NHI has the power to apply strategic health purchasing or prospective payments to optimize effectiveness and efficiency of the NHI fund. The NHI can dictate prices of health care, drugs, and other medical supplies from public and private health care providers. Hence, a single-payer NHI has strong power to make health system efficient.

3. A single NHI provides uniform procedures and benefits for everybody in the countries ensuring optimum social justice [7, 31]. These uniform procedures create less laborious efforts to educate the public. People who used the benefits can be good agents to make other people know how to utilize the benefits. This scheme provides efficient administration system because everybody and every health care provider will use a standardized system. Claim procedures can be organized using a single standard mechanism creating a very efficient system.

4. A single NHI provides economic incentives for health care providers to expand the care in areas where previously there is a shortage of private healthcare providers if the prices set by the NHI meet the production costs. So, the government or regional governments do not need to worry about establishing new hospitals.

5. All health care uses and the claim payments can be recorded in a single database and trend of health care utilization effects of medical procedures or drugs, side effects, and pattern of health-seeking behavior can be observed. This huge database could facilitate a ton of clinical and implementation research.

6. The prices and procedures of procurements of medical supplies and drugs can be standardized. Indonesia develops e-Catalog system where pharmaceutical companies and medical suppliers openly bid with lower prices and high volume across the country. Industries will be willing to lower the prices of their product for high volume. In addition, open and transparent competition will further induce efficiency of the industries. Pharmaceutical industries selling patent drugs can negotiate and deal with innovative financing to supply a high volume of their products.

7. The administrative costs of running a single NHI become very small compared to high revenue and multi-payer systems. Certainly, the NHI has very low

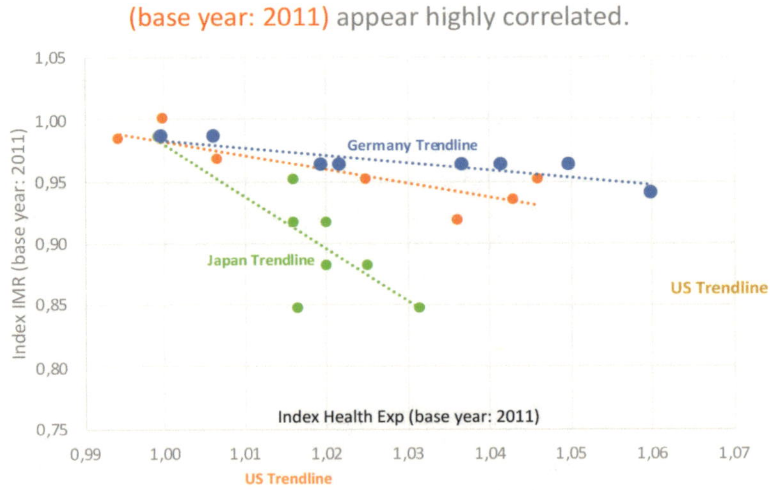

Figure 1.
Illustration of the correlation between index changes in health care expenditure (% GDP) with index changes in IMR of three countries between 2011 and 2017. 2011 index = 1.

Countries	Year	Public finance for health, % GDP	Infant mortality rate	UHC index* 2019
US—Multiple CHI dominance	2011	7.9	6.10	> = 80
	2012	7.9	6.00	
	2013	8.0	6.00	
	2014	8.3	5.90	
	2015	8.5	5.80	
	2016	8.6	5.80	
	2017	8.6	5.70	
UK—NHS single	2011	7.1	4.3	> = 80
	2012	7.0	4.1	
	2013	7.8	4.0	
	2014	7.8	3.9	
	2015	7.7	3.8	
	2016	7.8	3.8	
	2017	7.6	3.8	
Australia—NHS single	2011	5.9	3.8	> = 80
	2012	5.9	3.6	
	2013	5.9	3.5	
	2014	6.1	3.4	
	2015	6.4	3.3	
	2016	6.3	3.2	
	2017	6.3	3.2	
Italy—NHS single	2011	6.8	3.3	> = 80
	2012	6.8	3.2	
	2013	6.8	3.1	
	2014	6.8	3	
	2015	6.7	3	
	2016	6.6	2.9	
	2017	6.5	2.8	
Spain—NHS single	2011	6.7	3	> = 80
	2012	6.5	2.9	
	2013	6.4	2.8	
	2014	6.4	2.8	
	2015	6.5	2.7	
	2016	6.4	2.7	
	2017	6.3	2.7	

Countries	Year	Public finance for health, % GDP	Infant mortality rate	UHC index* 2019
Japan—NHI single	2011	8.9	2.3	> = 80
	2012	9.1	2.2	
	2013	9.1	2.1	
	2014	9.1	2.1	
	2015	9.2	2	
	2016	9.1	2	
	2017	9.2	1.9	
Korea—NHI single	2011	3.7	3.4	> = 80
	2012	3.7	3.3	
	2013	3.8	3.2	
	2014	3.9	3.1	
	2015	4.0	3	
	2016	4.2	2.9	
	2017	4.4	2.8	
Germany—SHI multiple	2011	8.1	3.4	> = 80
	2012	8.1	3.4	
	2013	8.3	3.3	
	2014	8.4	3.3	
	2015	8.5	3.3	
	2016	8.6	3.3	
	2017	8.7	3.3	
France—SHI multiple	2011	8.5	3.1	> = 80
	2012	8.6	3.1	
	2013	8.7	3.1	
	2014	8.9	3.1	
	2015	8.8	3.2	
	2016	8.8	3.2	
	2017	8.7	3.3	

**Coverage of essential health services (defined as the average coverage of essential services based on tracer interventions that include reproductive, maternal, newborn and child health, infectious diseases, non-communicable diseases and service capacity and access, among the general and the most disadvantaged population). The indicator is an index reported on a unitless scale of 0 to 100.*

Table 2.
Comparison of Public Finance as % GDP and IMR of Some Developed Countries with different health financing Schemes 2011–2018. Processed from World Bank Data and UHC Monitor 2021.

administrative expenses compared to CHI, which can absorb up to 25% of the total premium income. The administrative costs of NHI in Asia ranged from 1.8% in Taiwan to about 4% in Indonesia. Most Medicare programs in the US, Canada, and Australia also consume less than 4% of revenue. The average administrative expenses of the German's sickness funds were also around 4% of the total revenues.

8. When the NHI already reaches its maturity, providing quality health care to all populations with no catastrophic health spending, the NHI can be national pride.

If we consider tax-funded NHS as also a single payer with the government as the payer, this single-payer system or tax-funded system also has the above advantages. Evidence shows that countries applying NHS model, such as the UK, Nordic countries, Italy, and Spain, spent less than 10% of their GDP to achieve universal health coverage. In contrast, the US with dominance CHI has spent above 16% of its GDP in the last 10 years with relatively similar health outcomes with those developed countries with NHS or single-payer NHI.

As an illustration, in **Figure 1** we plot the index of health expenditures and infant mortality rates of three countries using 2011 as the base (index =1) and trend of decreasing IMR up to 2017. We use the World Bank data to illustrate the correlation between changes in health expenditures per capita and changes in IMR of Germany (blue dots), Japan (green dots), and the USA (orange dots). The figure illustrates that a virtual (quasi) single-payer health financing system in Japan had better performance in decreasing IMR with the same increase (change of index) from 2011 to 2017. Although this figure may not depict causal relationship, we can see the correlation is noted to be explored more.

We also provide **Table 2** illustrating the same level of UHC Index of high-income countries, public health spending as % GDP, and IMR per 1000 live births from 2011 to 2017. Data from the World Bank and the UHC Monitoring is used to develop this table.

6. Conclusion and recommendation

To ensure UHC and equitable access of at least essential health care for everyone in a country, public financing for health is absolutely needed. Public finance for health using single-payer scheme has a lot of advantages yielding more effective and more efficient financing schemes. Tax-funded, NHS model, or single-payer NHI model appears to be more effective and more efficient to produce expected outcomes of IMR. Multiple payer system of SHI appears somehow less effective and less efficient compared to the single-payer, monopsonist system. The authors recommend that LMICs that have not achieved UHC and are under consideration to reform health financing system may explore the possibility of introducing a single-payer health financing system. If a tax-funded (NHS) model is not possible, implementing SHI gradually to achieve an NHI would be a preferred choice. However, political battles need to be anticipated.

Conflict of interest

We do not have any conflict of interest. No fund from external authors is used for this chapter.

Notes/thanks/other declarations

None.

Author details

Hasbullah Thabrany* and Mutia Sayekti
The Indonesian Health Economist Association, Jakarta, Indonesia

*Address all correspondence to: hasbullah.thabrany@gmail.com

References

[1] Saksena P, Smith T, Tediosi F. Inputs for universal health coverage: A methodological contribution to finding proxy indicators for financial hardship due to health expenditure. BMC Health Services Research. 2014;**14**(1):1-10

[2] WHO. Tracking Universal Health Coverage: 2021 Global monitoring report [Internet]. Who.int. 2022. Available from: https://www.who.int/publications-detail-redirect/9789240040618. [Accessed: May 31, 2022]

[3] UK Department of Health. The NHS Constitution, the NHS belongs to us all. [Internet]. 2022. Available from: https://assets.publishing.service.gov.uk/government/uploads/system/uploads/attachment_data/file/170656/NHS_Constitution.pdf. [Accessed: April 23, 2022]

[4] Wagstaff A, Eozenou P, Smitz M. Out-of-pocket expenditures on health: A global stocktake. The World Bank Research Observer. 2020;**35**(2):123-157

[5] Financial Protection [Internet]. Who.int. 2022. Available from: https://www.who.int/health-topics/financial-protection#tab=tab_1. [Accessed: April 23, 2022]

[6] Evans R. Strained Mercy. Toronto: Butterworths; 1984

[7] Vaughn EJ, Vaughn TM. Fundamental Risk and Insurance. 11th ed. USA: Willey & Sons; 2013. p. 686

[8] Pitacco E. The individual perspective: The need for health insurance. Health Insurance. 2014:1-10

[9] Ghosh B. Rich doctors and poor patients: Market failure and health care systems in developing countries. Journal of Contemporary Asia. 2008;**38**(2):259-276

[10] World Health Organization. Earmarked Tobacco Taxes: Lessons Learnt from Nine Countries. Geneva: The No Tobacco unit (TFI), Department of Health Promotion, WHO; 2016

[11] American Health Insurance Plans. Fundamental Health Insurance, Part A. Washington DC: American Health Insurance Plans; 2011

[12] Thabrany H. Jaminan Kesehatan Nasional. Jakarta: Rajagrafindo Ltd; 2015. p. 394

[13] Gruber L, Shadle M, Polich C. From movement to industry: The growth of HMOs. Health Affairs. 1988;7(3):197-208

[14] World Bank Group. Global Economic Prospects. Washington DC: The World Bank; 2022. p. 4

[15] Karaca-Mandic P, Abraham JM, Phelps CE. How do health insurance loading fees vary by group size?: Implications for Healthcare reform. International Journal of Health Care Finance Economy. 2011;**11**(3):181-207. DOI: 10.1007/s10754-011-9096-4

[16] World Health Organization. Regional Office for the Western Pacific. 2015. The Kingdom of Thailand health system review. WHO Regional Office for the Western Pacific. Available from: https://apps.who.int/iris/handle/10665/208216

[17] Tikkanen R, Osborn R, Mossialos E, Djordjevic A, Wharton GA. International Health Care System Profiles Germany. Germany [Internet]. Commonwealthfund.org. 2022. Available from: https://www.commonwealthfund.

org/international-health-policy-center/countries/germany. [Accessed: May 16, 2022]

[18] KPMG. Individual Income Tax Rates Table. [Internet]. 2022. Available from: https://home.kpmg/xx/en/home/services/tax/tax-tools-and-resources/tax-rates-online/individual-income-tax-rates-table.html. [Accessed: April 24, 2022]

[19] Busse R, Blümel M, Knieps F, Bärnighausen T. Statutory health insurance in Germany: A health system shaped by 135 years of solidarity, self-governance, and competition. The Lancet. 2017;**390**(10097):882-897

[20] Normand C, Busse R. Social health insurance financing. Europe. 2002;**59**:59-79

[21] NHIS Korea. National Health Insurance System of Korea. Seoul: NHIS Korea; 2015

[22] Ministry of Health and Welfare Taiwan, ROC. National Health Insurance Annual Statistical Report 2019. Taipei, 2019

[23] Philippine Health Insurance Corporation. Universal Health Care: Trailblazing a new era of quality health care. Phil Health 2019 Annual report, Manila, 2020

[24] [Internet]. 2022. Available from: https://japanhpn.org/en/hs1/. [Accessed: April 24, 2022]

[25] Savedoff WD, Smith AL. Achieving Universal Health Coverage: Learning from Chile, Japan, Malaysia and Sweden. Washington, DC: Results for Development Institute; 2011

[26] Tatar M et al. Turkey health system review. European Observatory. 2011;**13**:43-44

[27] Lan JY-C. Achieving and sustaining Universal Health Coverage: Fiscal reform of the National Health Insurance in Taiwan. Applied Health Economics and Health Policy. 2016;**15**(6):717-731

[28] Busse R, Schwartz FW. Philippines' National Health Insurance Act. The International Journal of Health Planning and Management. 1997;**12**(2):131-148

[29] Kwon S. Thirty Years of National Health Insurance in South Korea: Lessons for achieving Universal Health Care Coverage. Health Policy and Planning. 2008;**24**(1):63-71

[30] Petrou P, Samoutis G, Lionis C. Single-payer or a multipayer health system: A systematic literature review. Public Health. 2018;**163**:141-152

[31] Hsiao WC, Cheng S-H, Yip W. What can be achieved with a single-payer NHI system: The case of Taiwan. Social Science and Medicine. 2019;**233**:265-271

Chapter 3

Health Insurance for Economically Disadvantaged People in LMICs: What are the Best Options?

Samuel George Anarwat

Abstract

The choice of a health care financing system can have both good and unintended devastating consequences on access to and delivery of quality affordable universal health care of a country. This paper aims to explore successful factors of health insurance schemes and health policies that will ensure universal health coverage (UHC). The chapter explores equity or fairness as defined by the theory of justice to elucidate why there tend to be inequities in health insurance coverage. It proposes measures that could be adopted to ensure social health protection and financial sustainability of health financing schemes to achieve universal health coverage in low- and middle-income countries (LMICs). Good health is an essential capital good for promoting well-being and longevity, and quality health care is a derivative of good health among other social and economic determinants of health. Universal health insurance schemes provide financial risk protection for many population groups, especially the less privileged, against catastrophic episodes of illness and injury. However, inequities in health care are pervasive and have impoverished many because of catastrophic health care expenditures. Health insurance based on solidarity and progressive tax financing system with premium exemptions for the vulnerable, might be best for LMICs.

Keywords: health insurance, social health insurance, universal health coverage, low- and middle-income countries, equity, social justice, health care financing systems financial risk protection

1. Introduction

Good health is an important capital good for well-being and longevity [1], and quality health care is a derivative of good health among other social and economic determinants of health [2]. Universal health insurance schemes provide financial risk protection for many population groups, especially the poor, against catastrophic episodes of illness and accidents. However, inequities in health care are pervasive and have impoverished many because of excessive health care expenditures.

The choice of health care financing systems can have good or unintended devastating consequences on access to and delivery of quality affordable universal health care. Several countries in low- and middle-income countries (LMICs) are exploring and developing different health care financing mechanisms to pay for health care for the poor, while advanced nations are proposing new methods, revising, or reviving their health financing policies to ensure equitable and sustainable health care for all. These efforts are imperative because access to health care is a fundamental human right. However, unfair national health policies have left millions of people, especially the poor with no or scarce access with low quality. Those who are fortunate to have access do not have the expected quality when and where they need it. The Alma Ata declaration of universal health care, and "Health for All by the year 2000", though achieved some increase in anticipated health care. The Millennium Development Goals Policy and its targets were very good international public health financing strategies, but many developing countries could not achieve the set targets because of inequities in funds to implement the proposed strategies. Notwithstanding the difficulties in funding and other challenges, there were some improvements in global health status indicators.

Today, the global health community has set itself to achieve universal health coverage (UHC) through Goal 3 and Goal 6 of the United Nations' Sustainable Development Goals (SDGs), also known as the agenda 2030 [3]. These two goals, among others, seek to achieve universal health care for everyone, located everywhere, with all ages without discrimination in terms of financial ability to pay. Goal 6 that is directly linked to Goal 3 seeks to provide sufficient water and sanitation for all global communities (www.sustainabledevelopment.un.org).

Again, I hypothesize that this policy of universal health coverage would not also be realized unless there is concerted effort to ensure fair financing strategies, adequate funding for its implementation, and efficient monitoring systems to reduce corruption and duplication of financial resources. The paper further inquires into selected best choices and methods that will ensure efficient and sustainable health financing in LMICs. The concept of health insurance, health equity, examples of best practice health financing models, success factors, and red flags of selected health financing systems are illustrated in this paper. The impact of coronavirus-19 (COVID-19) on health systems financing in LMICs is also elaborated in this chapter.

2. Concept of health insurance

In the past, people would pay for their health care just as they would buy a shirt in the market. Thus, they would pay out-of-pocket (OOP) for their health care. This mode of financing health care is largely outmoded, but poverty, poor health care systems, and policy compel many countries to finance health care by OOP. Financing health care through these direct OOP can impoverish countless households, especially in LMICs. Health insurance can solve the problem of OOP in most poverty endemic countries.

Health insurance is a system of financing health care through resource mobilization and risk pooling where risk-averse individuals prepay some amount of money into a pool for future health care benefits. Using the principle of large numbers, a third party manages the pool and purchases health care for members (the insured) in the case of illness. For the pool of funds to grow substantially to serve the interests of members, there must be large numbers of individuals collectively contributing equitable amount of money into the financial resource pool and sharing their financial risk to enjoy the collective financial protection.

To sustain the financial pool, there must be cross-subsidization across all the members contributing to the health insurance pool. In the spirit of fairness, there must be established policy measures to ensure that the rich pays more and the poor pays less, each pays according to their abilities (proportion of their income) into the health insurance fund; also, the healthy pays for the sick and economically healthy people pay for children and elderly. It is important to, however, check adverse selection in the risk and resource pooling process.

Adverse selection in health insurance is a situation where majority of health risk persons, people with preexisting health conditions, vulnerable population such as children, aged persons, and women are those mostly registered in the health insurance scheme, while healthy people enroll less in the insurance scheme. When this adverse selection of members occurs in a health insurance scheme, the likelihood of it collapsing is very high. The reason is that utilization of health care tends to increase, and claims cost also increases above revenue, unless there are huge subsidies from the government or philanthropic organizations to supplement the revenue stream of the organization to offset the catastrophic health care expenditures.

In addition to adverse selection, two forms of moral hazards are very common in health insurance that are worth mentioning under concepts of health insurance: consumer and provider moral hazard.

Consumer moral hazard means that the individual alters his or her behavior inappropriately to benefit from the health insurance scheme. For example, the individual could impersonate with someone else's insurance card to obtain health care. When the hospital authorities are not very vigilant, the insurance member could also intentionally seek health care unnecessarily just because the person is insured and has not falling ill or gotten an accident to make a health claim.

However, in developing countries, and selected advanced countries, like Canada and United Kingdom where there is waiting time to see a physician, especially, the medical specialists which take very long time, no rational individual would want to wait in the long line for no apparent sickness or health condition, just because of being insured.

Provider moral hazards emanate from the health care organizations or health professional to unduly benefit from the health insurance of patients. Providers alter their behaviors to "cheat" the health insurance system to make supernormal profits. There is a huge perception that the health insurance fraud in advanced countries is an albatross in the health care financing system. Provider moral hazards are facilitated by the information asymmetry that health care providers or health care professionals wield. They can use the information asymmetry to manipulate the health insurance system to make additional money. Information asymmetry arises because health care professionals are the vital repository of knowledge of the health condition and treatment regime of the patients and can therefore manipulate the information to their (providers') advantage. For instance, if the health specialist decided to admit a patient on a health condition for 10 days instead of 5 days, the patient, though has the right to reject the number of days of the hospitalizations, does so at his or her own peril.

3. Methods of financing health care

The World Health Organization (WHO) defines health financing as the "function of a health system concerned with the mobilization, accumulation and allocation of money to cover the health needs of the people, individually and collectively, in the health system ... .. The purpose of health financing is to make funding available, as well as to set the right financial incentives to providers, to ensure that all individuals have access to effective public health and personal health care" [4].

Health care can be financed through various methods, including resource pooling through health insurance, out-of-pocket payments, and public finance through direct or indirect taxes.

Health care financing can be classified into three different typologies: private health insurance (PHI), social health insurance (SHI), and national health insurance (National Health Service) [5]. Both government and third-party payers, as in organized private health insurance schemes or government agencies, play an especially key role in purchasing and pooling risk. The choice of the financing mechanism would depend on numerous factors, including the political economy of health, the political ideology of the country, equity principle, social solidarity, economics and financial strength of the country, and organization of the social and economic structure of the country, including labor unions, financial systems, health systems, and political systems of governance [5]. The choices made are associated with various advantages and disadvantages. It suffices to say that there is no perfect system, and there is no blueprint for each country. There can be a mix of both Beveridge and "Bismarckian" health care financing systems. There are no pure Beveridge or Bismarck systems. The choice of health financing system, to the best of my knowledge, will depend, to a considerable extent, on the health financing goals and several variables of the country in question. Selected methods of health financing and payment methods and governance of health care financing schemes are discussed in the following section.

As already stated, different countries have different methods of financing health care. The most common methods include but not limited to:

3.1 Free medical care (usually financed by progressive direct taxes)

With this system, every resident of a country is covered by the health care system and receives free medical care irrespective of income level or type of employment. The government pays for the entire cost of the health care, the cost of health professionals, and health infrastructure. In theory, this system is equitable, provided there are strong monitoring mechanisms put in place to ensure quality of care, and there is a large and consistent source of government revenue allocation to the health sector. Most developing countries practiced the free medical systems in the 1950s to late 1970s, but it was not sustainable because dwindling government revenue and quality of care were questionable [5, 6].

3.2 Social health insurance (SHI)

Social health insurance scheme is another method of health care financing through compulsory or voluntary health insurance. Ghana's National Health Insurance Scheme (NHIS), for instance, is a combination of mandatory NHIS Levy, mandatory social security contribution of formal sector workers, and voluntary premium payment by the informal sector workers. In the case of compulsory social health insurance, all citizens contribute a prepayment determined by the terms and conditions of the scheme either based on income or through employment or flat sum, or through direct or indirect taxes. In turn, members of the social health insurance scheme benefit through the insurance coverage for their health care. With (private) voluntary social health insurance (as in the case of mutual health insurance schemes of Senegal and Ghana in the early stages of the introduction of health insurance), the underlying principle is solidarity, where members voluntarily contribute a premium to a pool for risk sharing and financing of their health care needs [7]. Social health insurance scheme can be an equitable way of financing health care with the employed when premiums are based on income and determined by the ability to pay. However, with the unemployed the government must pay premiums for the poor, vulnerable, and unemployed. This affords both the poor and the rich to contribute their respective quotas to the health insurance fund to ensure a buildup of large numbers and large pool of resources. In this case, there is a large pool of financial resources to ensure financial risk protection and sustainability of the scheme, all things being equal. The German social health insurance scheme (SHI) with substitutive private health insurance scheme (PHI) is worth emulating in LMICs, because it has stood the test of time and all odds for over 100 years with near universal coverage of the population and with sustainable quality health care. A snapshot of the German SHI is given in the following section. Germany was the first country in Europe (may be in the world) to establish SHI with substitutive PHI in Europe, in 1883, by Chancellor Otto Von Bismarck. The German SHI is dubbed the "Bismarckian" SHI system, attributed to Chancellor Bismarck. The main takeout of the scheme is that is backed by a strong legislation which makes it mandatory for both employees and employers. It is based on strong solidarity principle with members. Both employees and employers pay equal share of premium (50% employee and 50% employer contribution) to finance the SHI. Also, employees pay 14.7% of total gross income toward the SHI. The scheme is very democratic in terms of organization and governance and has disintegrated service providers throughout the country. The German SHI is one of the most sustainable SHI systems in the world which is worth replication in other countries. The key principles and success factors of the German SHI are summarized in **Table 1**.

The dual system of health insurance (SHI and PHI) enhances coverage of the population. In Ghana, Nigeria, and Senegal, like many LMICs, the health insurance systems are hybrid and enrollment are voluntary. But in Ghana, for instance, the enrollment in PHI is very insignificant due to the high premiums of private health insurance.

Most LMICs including Ghana, Nigeria, Rwanda, Uganda, and Thailand, and high-income countries such as Canada, Germany, the Netherlands, and Switzerland, among others have adopted the social health insurance model and are at various stages of achieving universal health coverage. Germany, for instance, is well known for the "Bismarckian" social health insurance health system, which has existed and provided quality health care for citizens and residents over 100 years, using the dual model: SHI with PHI. As already stated, the German SHI is worth replicating in LMICs and even other advanced countries.

3.3 Universal health insurance coverage (UHC)

"UHC means that all individuals and communities receive the health services they need without suffering financial hardship. It includes the full spectrum of essential,

Success factors	Challenges
• First country to establish SHI in Europe, in 1883, by Chancellor Otto Von Bismarck. • SHI backed by strong legislation • SHI sustained over a century. • Uninterrupted development and reforms of the SHI system. • Strong principle of solidarity among members. • Continuous coexistence of statutory health insurance (SHI) and substitutive private health insurance (PHI). • Provision of universal health coverage. • Free choice of sickness funds to enroll in SHI. • Free choice of PHI to enroll. • Equal employee and employer contribution in SHI premiums. • Mandatory SHI (more population coverage – about 87%. • PHI coverage (the rich – only about 11%). • Self-governance. • More sickness funds than PHI. • Decentralized health systems governance.	• Complex health systems governance. • Decentralized health systems governance can stifle decision-making in the SHI • Health care sectors are subject to different legislations. • Health care sectors are separated in terms of governance, financing, and reimbursement. • Fragmented health service provision. • Quality assurance and coordination across are of continuous grave concern to health policy. • Lack of integrated health information, a concern to health policy.

Analyzed from.

Table 1.
Key principles and success factors of the German SHI.

quality health services, from health promotion to prevention, treatment, rehabilitation, and palliative care across the life course" [8].

Universal health insurance coverage ensures that every resident of a country has health insurance coverage, either financed through social security contribution or tax financing as in the case of United Kingdom, New Zealand, and Sweden, among others, with varying degrees of implementation structures. Everyone pays through different forms of taxation, irrespective of the risk burden of the individual. This system of financing ensures equity in financing because members pay for their health care through different forms of taxation based on their incomes and are provided universal health coverage. However, it should be noted that universal health coverage has different dimensions and usually covers the entire population but may not cover all health care services. Also, it may not be completely free at the point of use. Members may subscribe to supplementary health insurance schemes to cover expensive services that may not be covered under the universal health scheme or pay out-of-pocket, as in the case of France. Universal health coverage is also a sustainable way of financing health care as tax payment is compulsory. The caveat is when the tax is regressive which can perpetuate inequities. The question that remains is whether members of the universal health insurance scheme may receive quality health care, where and when needed, without a long waiting time to see specialist health professional.

3.4 Private health insurance

Private health insurance (PHI) is an alternative mechanism of financing health care for populations. PHI schemes are independent private entities usually established to provide health care for populations usually for profits. Profit is the main motive of PHI schemes [9]. PHI is both a "bad" and a "good" in the sense that it provides both challenges and opportunities for the attainment of universal health coverage goals. Many LMICs have a combination of PHI and public or social health insurance schemes as part of their health financing systems, as in the case of Ghana, Nigeria, Uganda, Rwanda, Kenya, La Cote d'Ivoire, and Senegal, among others. The choice of private or public health insurance scheme as a health financing system policy has consequences. Countries like the United States, France, Germany, Canada, the United Kingdom, Ireland, and Switzerland have different forms and policies of PHI schemes, providing choices and health coverage for distinct categories of populations. Private health insurance usually thrives well in high-income countries, though, not without challenges.

PHI in the United States, for instance, is organized in different forms: a) employer-based health insurance plans through employee-employer contribution, b) direct purchase of insurance, where the individual buys health insurance direct from the private health insurance companies, or through a state or federal marketplace, and c) private health insurance for uniform service [10].

Germany operates a substitutive PHI the for the rich, alongside the mandated social health insurance as far back as the nineteenth century (1883) known as the Bismarckian Health System. Although, there is opportunity for members of the SHI to opt out to join the PHI, there are legal restrictions for opting out of the SHI for the private health insurance once enrolled, to protect the social health insurance scheme.

It is important to note that PHI is based on voluntary enrollment and can contribute to huge uninsured populations, especially if the cost of PHI is not regulated by the state to make it affordable, especially for the poor. Usually, PHI premiums are actuarially determined making the premiums expensive for less privilege health care consumers to afford. Private health insurance can contribute to large uninsured populations, especially in LMICs, and even in certain advanced countries like United States. In the Netherlands, for example, the state subsidizes those who are unable to pay for health insurance. In Ghana, the poor and the vulnerable are covered under the social net premium exemptions program. PHI in Ghana, though optional, is expensive and benefits mostly rich people. Arguments for and against PHI are illustrated in **Table 2**.

The dual system of health insurance (SHI and PHI) enhances the coverage of the population. In Ghana, Nigeria, and Senegal, like many LMICs, the health insurance systems are hybrid and enrollment are voluntary. But in Ghana, for instance, the enrollment in PHI is very insignificant due to the high premiums.

Most LMICs including Ghana, Nigeria, Rwanda, Uganda, Thailand, and high-income countries such as Canada, Germany, the Netherlands, and Switzerland, among others have adopted the social health insurance model and are at various stages of achieving universal health coverage. Germany, for instance, is well known for the "Bismarckian" social health insurance health system, which has existed and provided quality health care for citizens and residents over 100 years and still thriving.

3.5 Community-based health insurance (CBHI)

Despite the call for health care financing through health insurance by the WHO since 2010, and the recent commitment through the UN Sustainable Development Goals (Goal 3 and its targets) for universal health coverage, out-of-pocket spending still accounts for large proportions of total health spending in LMICs. For reasons

Arguments for PHI	Arguments against PHI
1. Best model in terms of providing efficiency and quality health care. 2. Reduces public health sector costs and expenditure. 3. PHIs have the capacity to finance and find solutions to public health systems challenges in the public sector. 4. Competition in the private sector (PHI sector) coupled with profit motives can enhance efficiency, quality of care, and reductions in costs of care. 5. PHI markets are innovative, dynamic, and more sensitive and responsive to health care consumer needs than public sectors. 6. Additional funding sources to complement public health services. 7. Provides alternatives for the haves.	1. In LMICs, PHI is mostly operated in the cities for the benefits of the privilege. 2. There are barely private pharmacy shops in rural areas in LMICs. 3. Have no capacity to deliver equitable health care services. 4. Not able to efficiently manage health care costs, raising grave equity concerns. 5. High administrative costs and unhealthy competition can lead to high health care costs which are usually transferred to health care consumers. 6. May affect incentives for growth in health expenditure and the production of health. 7. Mere demand and supply interplay imbalances coupled with information asymmetry can drive health care costs and perpetuate inequities in health care.

Analyzed from [11].

Table 2.
Arguments for and against PHI.

of inadequate financial mobilization capacity and fiscal space, many LMICs have adopted community-based health financing schemes (CBHIs) as alternative means of financing health care for financial risk protection. This informal sector mechanism of financing health care aims to reduce out-of-pocket payment for health care which can impoverish low-income households.

"Community-based health insurance is an umbrella term for the various types of community financing arrangements that have emerged because of high out-of-pocket spending, uncertainty surrounding anticipated financial flows from donors, and large and unregulated private sectors" (...) "CBHIS refers to prepayment plans that attempt to pool risks to reduce the financial risk an individual faces because of illness" [12–14].

The main distinguishing features of CBHI from other health insurance schemes are1) diverse groups of population coverage, 2) strong solidarity among members, 3) differentiated services in terms of benefits package, 4) variability in regulations and democratic governance, 5) different management styles, and 6) objectives. CBHI is not new in the global arena, but they are prevalent in sub-Saharan Africa. The classical examples are the "Mutuelles de Santé" (Mutual Health Organizations) in Senegal, Mali, Burkina, and Ghana in its formative stages of health insurance [6, 12, 14].

Ample evidence suggests that CBHI has been significant in providing financial protection and health care access to many rural and low-income populations. But, where premiums are somewhat high, affordability hampers access for the very poor in the community [8]. Notwithstanding, strong evidence suggest that that community-based health insurance (CBHI) provides some financial protection through reduction in out-of-pocket expenditure on health and enhance cost recovery. But there is little or no evidence on the effect of quality of health care and efficiency of care. In totality, the impact of CBHI on access to health care is insignificant [14].

CBHI schemes serve only a small section of the population and cannot be guaranteed as a measure for achieving universal health coverage. They can however set the pace as a complementary scheme to other more efficient systems of health financing such as national health insurance schemes [15].

Despite the strong contribution of CBHI in providing financial protection for members and some level of resource mobilization, the general effect is somewhat small. CBHI schemes are insignificant in reaching the very poor. Hence, CBHI is necessary but may not be sufficient solution for risk pooling and revenue mobilization for health care in LMICs because of low population coverage and fragmented groupings.

> *"Both theory and evidence suggest that the traditional CBHI model – relying only on voluntary, small-scale schemes with little or no subsidization of poor and vulnerable groups – can play only a limited role in helping countries move towards universal health coverage (UHC). CBHIs cannot be expected to provide a major source of funding or coverage, and hence can at best provide only a complementary role as part of a national health financing strategy toward UHC. This is partly because people with few health needs tend not to join on a voluntary basis, and there is usually little or no subsidization for poor and other vulnerable groups. Health service utilization rates of members, however, generally increase after enrollment" [15].*

Among other things, health insurance thrives on large numbers (risk pool) and sustainable revenue. However, with strong legislation and community solidarity, LMICs can merge CBHI schemes to form a single-payer national health insurance scheme, as in the case of Ghana and Rwanda. CBHI schemes can be a springboard for the establishment of national health insurance scheme in countries where they exist, but they may not ensure equity in access to health care and cross-subsidization of risks.

In the next section, the paper expounds on John Rawls' theory of justice and its linkages with equity in health care financing.

4. Rawls' theory of social justice

John Rawls denotes equity as social justice and fairness [16]. He argues that the main pillar of social justice is grounded on the basic social structure and the social institutional distribution of fundamental rights and duties. Consequently, the political institution and economic and social arrangements decide the division of advantages from social cooperations. Also, social structure is the central pillar of social justice because it is composed of diverse social strata. People are born into the society with different opportunities and different expectations which are often decided by the political systems, as well as economic and social determinants in life. This implies that social institutions are structured in such a way that provides advantages to some groups of the society than others. According to Rawls [16], these social inequalities from the onset become pervasive and affect individual's chances in life. Rawls, therefore, proposes the application of social justice to cure or remedy unavoidable inequalities (inequities) in the society.

In the context of health financing, thus, buying health insurance for the people, social justice must regulate the fundamental elements of the economic, social, and health system so that the distribution of health care is fair. Social justice must be the cardinal principle and the applied strategy to distribute the fundamental health rights, to ensure that both economic and social opportunities prevail in various parts of the society. Rawls recommends social justice and economic redistributive justice [16].

Contextualizing health care financing by social justice and equity lens, it means providing health insurance coverage to all without jeopardizing their livelihood.

It also implies providing both the insured and the uninsured the best quality health care with maximum respect and dignity. Additionally, it suggests that health care providers and political systems should eschew greed, avarice, and corruption, and instead, be transparent and accountable to provide equitable universal health coverage to all, everywhere, at the right time, right quantities, and quality.

The ideals of social justice connote the adoption of the universal health coverage principles to provide financial risk protection for all residents irrespective of their ability to pay or not. No one should be impoverished because of catastrophic health care costs, usually, out-of-pocket. Consequently, social institutions mandated to purchase health insurance should do so based on equity and social justice. The guiding principle of universal health coverage should be equity, thus, reducing avoidable unfairness in health care financing coverage and access.

5. Equity in health care financing

Equity has been one of the important variables in health care systems, but inequities in health care financing and access are still very pervasive. Ample evidence suggests that the poor have less access to health care and suffer more devasting consequences of morbidity and mortality than the rich. The poor have lower levels of health care utilization than the rich, though they have more health needs and spend more on health care as percentage of their income than the wealthy individuals [17].

In this section, equity is contextualized as equity in access to health insurance, health care, and equity in health care delivery: distribution of health care services, urban-rural dichotomy, and ethnic minority communities. The Nobel Prize winner Amartya Sen [18] argues that health is one of the most important variables of human life and an important constituent of human capability, but the pervasiveness of inequalities in health care access and delivery is more disturbing than any other sectors.

Equity in health means that ideally everyone should have a fair opportunity to invest in their health to attain full health potential without any one being disadvantaged from achieving this potential if it can be avoided [19]. Equity can, thus, be explained as an ethical concept which is grounded in the principles of distributive social justice. Regrettably, different people and different authorities tend to interpret equity in diverse ways. To counterbalance the open interpretation of equity and create an operational concept, Braverman and Gruskin [20] defined equity (in health) as "the absence of socially unjust or unfair health disparities, the absence of systematic disparities in health (or in the major social determinants of health) between social groups who have different levels of underlying social advantage/disadvantage." This definition reminds us that the society is composed by diverse groups of people with different capabilities, sexual orientation, and different wealth gradients with unique needs in various locations. We call for a society where both the haves and the have-nots have equitable health insurance and universal health coverage without discrimination.

Based on the experts' definitions and Rawls' theory of justice, I conceptualize equity in this paper, as fairness in financial contribution (premium payment), fairness in health insurance coverage and access to health care, fairness in health care delivery, and fairness in the determination of benefits package. For example, the premiums of health insurance should be based on individuals or households' ability to pay. The wealthy individuals or households should pay more, according to some progressive principle while poor pay less, and indigents should be covered by safety net insurance.

6. Sustainable health care financing

Financial sustainability of health care financing is explained based on WHO's sustainable health care financing framework [21]. The frameworks explain sustainability in health care financing as the inter-relationship between revenue mobilization, risk pooling for financial protection, and efficient purchasing to meet the needs for all. The sustainability goal requires that the three interconnected health financing system functions: revenue collection, financial and risk pooling, and purchasing of health care services are met. Additionally, health care services should be provided according to need, quality, opportunity, and dignity, regardless of individual's ability to pay [6]. Sustainable health care financing can be conceptualized as the best and efficient mechanisms of organizing three components of the health insurance functions to provide continuous health care to the population, explained as revenue mobilization.

6.1 Revenue mobilization

Revenue mobilization means the measures adopted to raise revenues from various sources, identification of funding sources, and collection methods to finance the health services as well as the provider payment mechanisms. Sustainability of health insurance scheme depends on the quantum of the funds raised and the efficient management of the funds.

6.2 Fund pooling

Fund pooling refers to policies established to build an advanced accumulated funding from various sources on behalf of the population. Pooling also means risk sharing between different people who have different incomes, ages, and illness risk.

6.3 Resource allocation and purchasing

Resource allocation and purchasing simply means paying providers health care services on behalf of the insured. It refers to the measures used to buy health care services from public and private providers for and on behalf of health care consumers.

These three financing functions interact at country health policy level and translate into mobilizing adequate and sustainable revenues in an efficient and equitable manner to provide individuals with the needed essential health services and financial risk protection against unforeseen catastrophic episode of illness or injury.

Effective and efficient combination of the health financing functions and the policies together, through the intermediate sustainability goals such as transparency and accountability, can yield a sustainable and resilient health financing system for a country.

7. Health financing schemes in LMICs, lesson from Ghana and Thailand

Since the adoption of the WHO's world health report in 2000, governments of LMICs have formulated strategies to finance health care to increase equity in access to health care in their respective countries. Despite the frantic efforts and success chalked by various countries in this direction, there are still rooms for improvements. Rwanda, for instance, has achieved near-universal health coverage, and Ghana, Nigeria, Senegal, and Tanzania have made giant strides in the establishment of national health insurance schemes. However, many countries in sub-Saharan Africa are at various stages of their health financing schemes. This section expounds on selected health financing schemes that have successfully been applied to cover all categories of individuals, including poor people to draw useful lessons for adaptation and replication in other peer countries. Ghana and Thailand are excellent examples of robust and successful health financing schemes worthy of emulation. These two countries present excellent best practices for replication, but not without challenges on their path to universal health coverage. The two countries' insurance schemes were chosen because of their uniqueness. The successes and challenges are elucidated in the following section.

7.1 Success factors and red flags of Ghana's National Health Insurance Scheme

Ghana's National Health Insurance Scheme (NHIS) was established in 2003 by an act of parliament (Act 650, 2003 [22], revised by Act 852, 2012 [23]) to provide equitable health care to all residents of Ghana. The NHIS was meant to be pro-poor recognizing the gap in health care between the poor and the rich in access to health. Funding of the scheme is tax-based (3.5%) which accounts for the National Health Insurance Levy, an indirect value-added tax on purchase of goods and services; it is also financed by a voluntary contribution (NHIS Premiums of the informal sector population GHS240 ($34.00, in 2022 exchange rate), and social security contribution (2.5%) applied to formal sector employees, and other financing sources such as grants, donations, and investments returns. It is worth noting that about 75% of the total NHIS funding is from NHIS Levy. The scheme has a comprehensive and generous benefits package covering closed to 90% of all diseases, health conditions, and accidents. However, major and complicated surgeries often may not be covered. Medications and prescribed drugs are covered, but most often there are limited supply of essential medication at the hospitals, and patients are given prescription paid out-of-pocket [6, 22, 23].

After almost two decades of its implementation, the scheme has still attained the required universal population coverage. Only about 50% of diverse groups of the population have enrolled in the NHIS, which raises the question why are the rest of the 50% not covered under the NHIS? What is not going right in the NHIS policies and strategies? Notwithstanding the challenges, the NHIS is considered a best practice scheme for replication on other African and other LMICs. In the following section, I analyze the success factors but also indicate the red flags of Ghana's NHIS. As much as these success factors can be replicated or adopted in other countries on their paths to health insurance, it is important to note that replication of these success factors in other LMICs should be done with caution in the cultural-specific and political context of the country. The underlying key factors that influence the success of Ghana's NHIS are illustrated in **Table 3**. The list is not exhaustive, as suggested by Anarwat and Shepard in 2020.

7.2 Thailand's universal health care coverage scheme (UCS)

Thailand's National Health Insurance Scheme (UCS) was established in 2001. The UCS is organized in three different forms of schemes: 1. Social Security Scheme

Success factors	Red flags
1. Strong political will.	1. Nonadherence to the gatekeeper system.
2. Appropriate legislation	2. Provider shopping on the part of NHIS members.
3. History of social solidarity	3. Provider moral hazards.
4. Tax funding	4. Corruption in the health delivery service.
5. Safety nets for the poor and vulnerable	5. NHIS provider collusion.
6. Good governance.	6. Provider moral hazards.
7. Decentralized local government system	7. Adverse selection.
8. Vibrant and well-structured health systems.	8. Paradox of exemptions policy.
9. The role of CHAG and mission hospitals	9. Inappropriate provider payment method.
10. Learning-by-doing approach	10. Controversy of NHIS capitation payment system.
11. Hospital user-fees ("Cash and Carry") policy challenges.	11. Delays in claims processing.
12. Multifaceted communication and marketing approach.	12. Undue political influences on the NHIS.
13. Development partners' support (technical and financial support).	13. Unrealistic premiums and low. Enrollment of the economically active population.
14. Comprehensive benefits package.	14. Poor quality health care services.
15. Very low-cost premiums.	15. Continuously low enrollment of the economically active populations in the informal sector.
16. Social Security and National Insurance Trust, Members' Contribution.	
17. Health insurance user portability.	
18. Academic and operational research	
19. Multiple providers and free choice of providers.	

Analyzed from [24].

Table 3.
Success factors and red flags of Ghana's NHIS.

(SSS) for private sector workers; 2. Civil Servants' Medical Benefits Scheme (CSMBS) for government employees, their spouses, dependents less than 20 years, and their parents; and 3. UCS for the rest of the population which aims to cover all the population not covered by the SSS, mostly informal sector workers.

The UCS has 99.8% population coverage. It is funded through a combination of taxes and contribution (premium) from members. This premium is exceptionally low, about 30 Baht ($1.00) the starting based level [25]. The success factors and challenges are illustrated in **Table 4**.

8. Impact of COVID-19 on health financing systems in LMICs

SARS-CoV-2 virus, a highly infectious and deadly disease, popularly known as coronavirus (COVID-19) after it was first reported in Wuhan, China, in 2019, has devasted global public health and global health systems. In a spate of 3 months, the disease took global leaders by surprise and spread through the world like wildfire, destroying health systems, wiped out populations in advanced and developing countries. COVID-19 caused panic, anxiety, and mental health challenges, devastated families, destroyed business, increased health care financing and delivery costs, and

Key success factors	Challenges
1. Established with low contribution –30 Baht ($1) copayment per out-patient (OPD) and in-patient visits. 2. Entirely tax-financed (copayment abolished in 2006). 3. Comprehensive benefits package focused on primary health care. 4. Covers preventive and health promotion services. 5. Capitation payment mechanism for OPD care. 6. Global budget system for diagnosis related groupings (DRGs) for in-patient care. 7. Strong political will – "30 baht can pay for all disease" campaign. 8. Foundational support by civil society groups and NGOs – campaign for universal health coverage. 9. Implemented "Social Protection floors" (SPFs) –ILO *(guaranteed access to essential health care and basic income security for children, persons of working age, and the aged)* 10. Strong legal and institutional frameworks.	1. Inequalities in the Thai health systems (unequal distribution of health personnel and facilities between urban and rural areas. 2. Differential benefits packages among the health insurance schemes. 3. Rising costs due to generous benefits packages, chronic diseases, and aging populations. 4. Inefficiencies in the local government administration of health systems leading to leakages and duplication of resources. 5. Financial sustainability challenges.

Analysis from [25].

Table 4.
Success factors of Thailand's universal health care coverage scheme.

brought down global travels to a near halt. Several cities in both advanced countries and LMICs experienced lockdowns for several months. For the first time in the history of the world, international and domestic flight in many countries were banned for more than a year, since COVID-19 was declared a global pandemic on March 11, 2019 by the World Health Organization (WHO).

On May 2, 2022, WHO reported a global total of COVID-19 infections stood at 511,275,451 COVID-19 cases and 6,238,320 deaths with a case fatality ratio (CFR) of 1.2% in 227 countries and territories. The reported cumulative cases (percentage of global cases) from the WHO regions except Africa were Eastern Mediterranean Region 18,377,400 (4%), European Region 215,216,599 (42%), Region of the Americas 153,175,779 (30%), South-East Asia Region 57,870,460 (11%), and Western Pacific Region 54,757,461 (11%). At the same period, a total of 11,453,205 COVID-19 cases and 252,165 deaths, with CFR of 2.2%, were reported by the 55 African Union (AU) Member States (MS). Although the incidence in Africa represents only 2% of all cases and 4% of all deaths reported globally, the impact on individual AU Member States was catastrophic. Forty (73%) of individual AU Member States reported CFRs higher than the global CFR [26].

The good news is that the collaborative scientific research which led to the production of vaccines with boosters in advanced countries, such as the United States, the United Kingdom, Germany, and Russia, among others, is expected to curtail the mortality rates of the pandemic and the impact. Unfortunately, LMICs are still struggling to produce their first COVID-19 vaccine, and therefore, must rely on the collective benevolence of advanced countries through the COVAC initiative to vaccinate their populations.

The evidence suggests that over 4.6 billion people constituting 58% of the global population have been fully vaccinated. But, only 17% of the total population of Africa was fully vaccinated, as of May 2022 [27], which could be attributed to inadequate vaccine supply, vaccine myths and hesitancies, funding and procurement issues, among other factors. The economies of many LIMCs experienced negative economic growth, and huge negative impact on their health systems are still recuperating since the outbreak of COVID-19. The impact of COVID-19 pandemic should be a wake-up call for LMICs to adopt measures to strengthen their health systems and make them resilient.

9. Discussion, conclusions, and recommendations

Inequities in health insurance coverage and access to health care between people with different incomes and wealth are pervasive in several LMICs. Based on Rawls' theory of social justice, there is unfairness in health insurance coverage of which the less privilege people in society, especially in LMICs, have always been disadvantaged. The paper explored the types of health insurance schemes and the choices LMICs policymakers can make to ensure equitable health care for all. It elucidated on successful factors of key health insurance schemes and health policies that can ensure universal health coverage for all without anyone left out. The question often posed by LMICs policymakers is which type of health insurance scheme to implement and what should be the strategic factors to adopt for success.

To answer the question which insurance model to choose, it is important to conclude that there is no blueprint for successful implementation of a health insurance scheme that will cover the poor. However, the review of the existing types of health insurance schemes shows that publicly taxed-financed health insurance schemes tend to cover and benefit the poor. Publicly financed single-payer national health insurance schemes, as in Ghana, Thailand, United Kingdom, and Canada, facilitate the achievement of universal health coverage than private health insurance schemes. However, they all have their ups and downs. Proponents of PHIs argue that they ensure freedom of choice of health insurance, efficiency, and quality of care. But in most cases, PHIs are limited to the privilege, are profit-oriented, and do not ensure equity in health insurance coverage [11].

Where there is multiplicity of private health insurance schemes of all forms, as in the case of the United States, the poor tend to suffer in terms of coverage because of high premiums [10]. It is argued that PHI breeds competition and enhances technological advancement in health care and therefore promotes the quality of care delivery [11]. But what is the point of quality of care where large majority of the population have no health insurance and find it difficult to access health care? PHI might not be a good option for LMICs striving to achieve UHC. At best, private health insurance can be encouraged as a supplementary insurance to cover for highly sophisticated health care services, while the government subsidizes for the poor to ensure equity of access. Where PHI is the health financing policy, the government should adopt measures to cover the poor through subsidies or premium exemptions.

Though it would be naïve to recommend a particular health insurance model for any country as the best model for replication, the "Bismarkian" model has stood the test of time of time and, therefore, worth replication in LMICs but with caution. The caveat might be the large informal sector in LMICs and high unemployment rates, which might be difficult to mandate insurance contribution through social security. Even though CBHI is a community initiative based on social solidarity, the evidence suggests that they do not have the capacity to mobilize large pools or revenue and risk, and they may not be able to ensure universal health coverage [15]. Consequently,

CBHIs might not be recommendable option for LMIC who are about to start universal health insurance scheme. In LMICs with high prevalence of CBHIs, it is imperative that governments legislate to merge them to form a single-payer national health insurance scheme.

Progressive tax-based health insurance schemes, in the case of Ghana and Thailand, present best practices that LMICs can adapt while marking the red flags to avoid on their pathways to universal health insurance coverages. It is crucial for LMICs to understand that there is no perfect health insurance scheme or straight jacket strategies for success. It all depends on the terrain and the dynamics of the political economy.

Both advanced and developing countries are continuously experimenting models for equitable and sustainable health financing for quality UHC. There is no straight jacket or blueprint method to achieve Universal Health Coverage. Nonetheless, to implement a viable and sustainable health financing systems for universal health coverage, the best health financing and organizational options should be derived from a broad spectrum of choices, including, but not limited to, private financing options, tax-based financing, social health insurance, single-payer system, and mixed models' health financing systems. The choice of health financing systems should be driven by prevailing social, economic, and political economy factors. Progressive taxed-based single-payer systems with strong mechanisms put in place to check that abuse and corruption would be a better option to cover the poor and to achieve UHC. It is imperative to implement policies that are preponderantly country context-specific and culturally acceptable to get the people's buy-in. We recommend LMICs to adopt and adapt the best practice models of health insurance schemes to suit their prevailing economic, social, political, and cultural situations. COVID-19 had a huge devastating impact on the economies of LMICs. Implicitly, it behooves on LMICS to invest in research, health systems strengthening, financing, and human resource for health to establish strong health sectors against such unanticipated epidemics and pandemics. More in-depth and further research is needed to look at the impact of COVID-19 on health systems financing of LMICs [28].

Author details

Samuel George Anarwat
School of Public Health, Department of Health Services Policy, Planning, Management and Economics, University for Development Studies, Tamale, Ghana

*Address all correspondence to: anarwat@gmail.com; ganarwat@uds.edu.gh

References

[1] Grossman M. On the concept of health capital and the demand for health. Journal of Political Economy. 1972;**80**:223-255. DOI: 10.1086/259880

[2] Donabedian A. The quality of care: How can it be assessed? JAMA. 1988;**260**(12):1743-1748. DOI: 10.1001/jama.1988.03410120089033

[3] United Nations. Transforming Our world, the 2030 Agenda for Sustainable Development. 2022. Available from: www.sustainabledevelopment.un.org. [Accessed: April 10, 2022]

[4] World Health Organization (WHO). World Health Reports. Geneva: Financing for Universal Health Coverage; 2010

[5] Dewar DM. Essentials of Health Economics. Sudbury, MA: Jones Bartlett Publishers; 2010

[6] Anarwat S. Ghana's National Health Insurance Model: Advancing Financial Risk Protection, Equity of health Care Access, and Financial Sustainability ProQuest. Ann Arbor Ph.D. Dissertation; 2018

[7] Normand C, Weber A, et al. Social Health Insurance: A Guide-book. Verlag fur Akademische Schriften; VAS, Ludwigstr. Bad Homburg v.d.H. Germany· 2009;12 d:61348. ISBN 978-3-88864-491-7

[8] WHO. Universal Health Coverage, What is it? 2021. Available from: https://www.who.int/news-room/fact-sheets/detail/universal-health-coverage-(uhc). [Accessed: May 24, 2022]

[9] Colombo F. Private Health Insurance in OECD Countries: The Benefits and Costs for Individuals and Health Systems, OECDDELSA/ELSA/WD/HEA. Ann Arbor Ph.D. Dissertation 2004

[10] Edward RB, Barnett JC, Upton RD. Health Insurance Coverage in the United States: 2018 Current Population Reports, P60-267(RV). USA: Department of Commerce; 2019

[11] Tapay N, Colombo F. "Private Health Insurance in the Netherlands. A Case Study", OECD Health Working Paper. Paris: OECD; 2004

[12] Atim C, Diop F, Etté J, Evrard D, Marcadent P, Massiot N. The Contribution of Mutual Organizations to Financing, Delivery, and Access to Health Care: Synthesis and Research in Nine West and Central African Countries. Bethesda, MD: Abt Associates, Partnerships for Health Reform Project; 1998

[13] Bennett S, Kelley AG, Silvers B. 21 Questions on CBHF: An Overview of Community-Based Health Financing. Bethesda, MD: Abt Associates, Partnerships for Health Reform Project; 2004

[14] Schieber G, Baeza C, Kress D, Maier M. Chapter 12. Financing HealthSystems in the 21st Century. In: Jamison DT, Breman JG, Measham AR, Alleyne G, Claeson M, Evans DB, Jha P, Mills A, Musgrove P, editors. Disease Control Priorities in Developing Countries. 2nd ed. Washington (DC): Disease Control Priorities Project; 2006

[15] WHO. Community-based health insurance. 2020. Available from: https://www.who.int/news-room/fact-sheets/detail/community-based-health-insurance-2020#:~:text=Community-based%20health%20insurance%2. [Accessed: May 21, 2022]

[16] Rawls J. A Theory of Justice. Cambridge MA: The Belknap Press of Harvard University; 1999

[17] Owen O'D, van Doorslaer E, Wagstaff A, Lindelow M. Analyzing Health Equity Using Household Survey Data: A Guide to Techniques and Their Implementation. Washington, DC: The World Bank; 2008

[18] Amartya S. Why health equity? Health Economics. 2002;**11**(8):659-666

[19] Whitehead M. The concepts and principles of equity of equity in health. International Journal of Health Sciences. 1992;**22**:429-445

[20] Braveman P, Gruski S. Theory and methods: Defining equity in health care. Journal of Epidemiology and Community Health. 2003;**57**:254-258

[21] Kutzin. A descriptive framework for country-level analysis of health care financing arrangement. Health Policy. 2001;**56**:171-204

[22] Republic of Ghana. Ghana's National Health Insurance Act, 650. 2003

[23] Republic of Ghana. Ghana's National Health Insurance Act, 852. 2012

[24] Anarwat SG, Shepard DS. Health Care Financing Reforms in Ghana: Key Lessons for Uganda and other LMICs. In: Basaza R, Namyalo PK, Mayora C, Shepard DS, editors. The Journey to Universal Health Insurance Coverage, What Are the Lessons for Uganda and Other LMICs? New York: Nova Science Publishers; 2020

[25] International Labour Organization (ILO). Universal Health-care Coverage Scheme, Thaniland, Social Protection in Action: Building Social Protection Floors. 2016. Available from: https//www.socialprotection.org/gimi/gess/ResourcePDF.action?resource.resourceld=54059. [Accessed: January 5, 2022]

[26] Africa Union. Outbreak Brief #120: Coronavirus Disease 2019 (COVID-19) Pandemic Date of Issue. Africa: CDC; 2022

[27] African Union Centers for Disease Control and Prevention (AU CDC 2022). Outbreak Brief #120: Coronavirus Disease 2019 (COVID-19) Pandemic Date of Issue: 3 May 2022. Available from: https://africacdc.org/download/outbreak-brief-120-coronavirus-disease-2019-covid-19-pandemic/ [Retrieved: May 30, 2022]

[28] World Economic Forum. Why Sub-Saharan Africa needs a unique response to COVID-19. 2020. Available from: www.weforum.org/agenda/2020/03/why-sub-saharan-africa-needs-a-unique-response-to-covid-19/. [Accessed: May 23, 2022]

Chapter 4

National Health Insurance, the Informal Sector, and Elements of a New Social Contract in the 2019 UHC Act of the Philippines

Maria Cristina G. Bautista

Abstract

This chapter explores the governance issues in the implementation of insurance coverage for the informal labour sector in the context of universal health coverage (UHC). The COVID-19 pandemic highlights the vulnerabilities of the informal sector that remain overlooked by employer health insurance and are not targeted by the government's cash transfer programmes for the poor. While universal health coverage may, on paper, assure every one of the basic minimum health care packages, issues of capturing subsidies for and availing of similar no user charges for the poor may be a Gordian knot before universal coverage is achieved. The chapter interrogates this issue as follows—firstly, we present key health financing features of the Philippine efforts to cover the informal sector in the national health insurance programme; and secondly, based on a concept approach, we analyse the elements of a social contract that may enhance or break down relationships in informal sector health insurance—with the market, bureaucratic and networks in health systems. Implications are drawn on the design of institutional arrangements to capture subsidies, contributions, and provider payments as part of a post-pandemic new normal of greater health security through the financing of health in the context of a social contract.

Keywords: informal sector, health insurance, Philippines, universal health coverage, new social contract

1. Introduction

This chapter examines health insurance systems from the perspective of how health insurance access can be expanded in environments characterised by high levels of informality in employment, relative unaffordability of premiums, low benefit or service levels, revealed preference for private health care, and high inefficiencies in the management of social health insurance funds. This type of environment is prototypical not only for the Philippines but for other low to middle-income countries. Informal labour markets present a challenge to health insurance systems as there is no employer to co-share premium payments, nor are they adequately covered in government subsidies extended for those considered poor through the means test. It is this gap that is often cited as 'the missing middle' in social health insurance systems' [1].

Assessments of health coverage for the informal sector examine demand and supply-side issues peculiar to the sector, such as willingness to pay and ability to pay, premium levels, and collection structures, including cost-sharing modalities and fund sustainability. This chapter takes on the perspective of understanding the institutional context, the nature of coordination arrangements required to 'fit' the informal sectors' conditions into social health insurance schemes or in reverse, structure systems to cater to social insurance schemes for the more unorganised groups.

Health insurance systems have two inherent features—information asymmetries and adverse selection. Yet social health insurance schemes often bypass these concerns in the development of schemes to cover the informal sector. Information asymmetry fosters moral hazard, whereby insurance status signals the choices on diagnostics or treatment and quality of services recommended by providers, described in standard textbooks [2]. Moral hazard happens when the insured takes more risks, such as unhealthy or incautious consumption behaviour (smoking, driving under the drugs, or alcohol influence) as a result of the risks being insured. Adverse selection is created when risk pools may be more attractive to sicklier individuals. Private health insurance is known to select lower-risk individuals. These features create the knowledge gaps to coordinate transactions and behaviour in the informal sector, thus limiting health insurance coverage. The promise of social health insurance or universal health coverage (UHC) is premised on greater financial protection in the face of health risks, a larger population coverage to spread risks, and wider sets of services or benefits covered. These pillars of UHC form its mandate, affecting interactions among stakeholders and thus creating operating pressures for programme implementation.

The Philippines launched its universal health care Act in 2020, following the approval of a fresh-minted law, Republic Act 11223 in February 2019. Implementation was set for January 2020, when the COVID-19 pandemic struck. This twin setback provides an opportunity for reflection on an institutional design that is more inclusive, efficient, equitable for greater health security.

2. Features of informal employment in the Philippines and the health insurance programme by PhilHealth for the informal sector

This section covers the estimates of the informal economy for the country, its features in terms of demographics, and some context.

2.1 The size and magnitude of informal employment

Using a proxy indicator[1] based on its labour force surveys, in the absence of a direct survey, the Philippine's Department of Labour and Employment (DOLE) representative to the Global Knowledge Sharing forum shared the statistics on the informal

[1] Since 2008, there has been no direct survey of the informal economy. During this 2008 Informal Sector Survey (ISS) 29.8 million workers were considered in informal employment or 75% of Filipino workers (WB 2010). Under proxy indicators, there were only 19.4 million informally employed workers considered in 2008, indicating an underestimation of the number of informal workers by nearly 10 million.

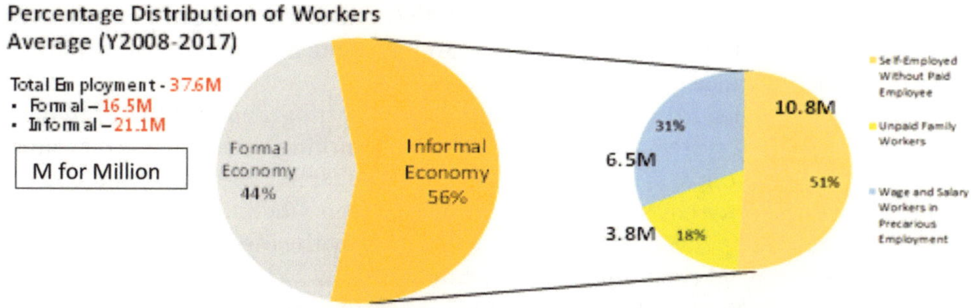

Source: Department of Labor and Employment (2018). *Size of the Informal Economy in the Philippines.*[4]

Figure 1.
Size of informal employment. Source: Department of Labour and Employment (2018). Size of the Informal Economy in the Philippines [3].

economy. **Figure 1** shows that from 2008 to 2017, there was an average of 21.1 million workers in the informal economy (estimated by the number of self-employed without paid employees, unpaid family workers, and wage and salary workers in precarious employment). This comprised 56% of the total employment; while workers in the formal economy (estimated by the employer in own family farm or business, and the wage and salary workers with the permanent job or business) were 44% of total employment or an average of 16.1 million workers. The figures include the agricultural sector. This figure of 56% of total employment as informal is relatively lower than the 68.2% regional average, with agriculture and China included, for the Asia and Pacific [4].

Out of the 21.2 million workers in the informal economy in the Philippines, in the 10-year average, the self-employed accounted for 10.8 million (51%), followed by wage and salary workers in precarious employment with 6.5 million (31%), and unpaid family workers with a total of 3.8 million (18%). In 2017, there were 17.62 million workers in formal employment and 22.68 million in informal employment. In the 10 years, informal employment grew by 16.5%.

Informality in employment is expected to increase due to the restrictions on movement and outright lockdown of workplaces and cities due to the pandemic. The Asian Development Bank reported that by January 2021, 1.7 million wage and salary jobs were lost and the informal sector numbers rose to 435 thousand. This was just one year from the start of the pandemic in 2020 [5]. Further surges in infections and movement restrictions as part of pandemic control are likely to see rising numbers of people getting off formal work in favour of more flexible arrangements. While informal work numbers indicated that there are estimated to be comprising the second quintile of families in the distribution of income, working arrangements particularly in the sharing economy sector, such as Uber, Grab drivers and online sellers will see the expansion of the informal sector towards the middle quintiles.

2.2 PhilHealth: the national health insurance corporation and its informal sector programme

The country's national health insurance program was instituted in 1995, with health funds carved out from the social security system for employed workers who paid in monthly contributions towards health, work accident, life insurance, and pensions since 1969. The Philippine Health Insurance Corporation (PhilHealth) absorbed and managed health insurance funds and progressively overtook other health insurance schemes, such as those for overseas Filipino workers for their families left behind, those covered by charitable agencies, and its name is synonymous with the national health insurance programme.

In the late 80s to 90s, Medicare, the health insurance programme attached to the private social security system (SSS), was involved in working with organised groups, mostly community groups, some on rotating savings schemes, who were enjoined to include health insurance coverage as a benefit to members. Technical assistance and material support for operating systems were provided by the Medicare programme, through the German aid programme (GTZ) called SHINE. When the Indigent Programme got into good momentum, many of the groups were incorporated in the LGU sponsorship, others closed.

PhilHealth instituted a voluntary contribution scheme in early 2012 targeting informal employment workers belonging to cooperatives or those organised through non-government organisations (NGOs) through the organised groups programme. The institution made various efforts to gather these groups, providing incentives to the savings associations, cooperative banks, or non-government organisations to collect funds from members, advance or loan members their premium payments in 2017. When group collectors were no longer willing to collect, organised member groups thus reverted to individually paying membership. It was reported in 2014 that dropout rates or regular non-payment of premiums were two-thirds of the membership in the individual economy scheme (as the informal sector programme has been renamed) [6].

PhilHealth has other member categories, aside from those in formal employment. The 'sponsored member' group is the largest, comprising 50% of membership in 2015. Sponsored members are those who enjoy full state or other state agencies' subsidies for premiums. The biggest group of sponsored members belongs to the beneficiaries of the government's conditional cash transfer (CCT) programme. In this cash transfer programme, a means test is utilised to target the deserving beneficiaries who are considered poor through 24 sets of proxy variables of income and well-being variables. Other sponsored members, including retirees and pensioners (aged over 60), are considered lifetime members and non-paying. Under the new UHC Act, sponsored members are fully protected by the no-balance-billing policy. This policy mandates that as long as there are public hospital wards available, these members cannot be charged with other expenses exceeding their PhilHealth benefits.

In 2015, sponsored members comprised 50% of PhilHealth membership, followed by 30% from the formal sector, 9.5% from the retirees or lifetime members. The balance, or around 10%, was from the informal and self-employed members. This share has gone up to 18% according to a 2020 study [7].

The idea of public-organised groups' partnerships in funds collection has been pioneering [6]. The problems related to the informal sector programme of PhilHealth can be traced to the following—(1) relatively unaffordable premiums for its target informal sector groups; (2) lack of systems to verify membership with contributions and thus smoothen authorisations at the time of use; (3) low level of benefits and substantial out-of-pocket expenses; (4) learning by doing approach that lacked consultation and evidence-based studies which led to policy confusion for implementors; and (5) a complex financial management system which made funds tracking unwieldy. PhilHealth experienced fund deficits arising from its expansion of coverage to other sponsored members, diversification to non-hospital-based benefits, and other fund management issues. The fund which reported a surplus for much of its existence [8] suffered deficits when subsidies overtook member payments as the dominant revenue source [9]. Media reported on anomalies involving the PhilHealth Board's authorisation of across-the-board payroll bonuses to employees. This was eventually ruled by the highest court to be illegal and without proper authorisation [10].

This assessment can apply to the whole PhilHealth programme; notwithstanding strides taken in continuing efforts to increase coverage and improve equity [11]. Benefits have been bolstered as well with the inclusion of other outpatient benefits, including costly procedures, such as dialysis and cataract operations, and catastrophic care packages, such as Z benefits [12]. These gains were obtained at the cost of financial weakening and other administrative setbacks, which caused delays in payment to providers and heightened the lack of trust and other credibility issues with stakeholders [13].

3. Conceptual underpinnings and related literature

In the light of the new UHC Act and the attention directed to the health sector due to the pandemic, a primordial question is raised. What is the appropriate governance structure framing a pluralistic health system often found in many low and middle-income countries (LMIC), such as the Philippines? From an economic organisation perspective, Williamson ([14], p. 673) viewed operationalising the concept of governance from 'the lens of a contract (rather than the neoclassical lens of choice)'. This perspective views the unit of analysis concerning the organisation problem not in terms of the individual but of the transaction. According to the early (mid-twentieth century) institutional economist, J. Commons, a contract 'must contain the three principles of conflict, mutuality and order' ([14], p. 673). This section extends the analysis of the organisation of national health insurance as a social contract problem, examining the nature of transactions in health care, the practice of rules, regulations, source(s) of organisational stability, and the relations with stakeholders fostered.

Commons' view of the contract contextualised in economic organisation lens as conflict-mutuality-order is similar to the impetus for the classical social contract. The work of early political philosophers, however, emanated from the perspective of *individuals* agreeing to a code of conduct, with the state's role as arbiter and enforcer. Loewe, Zintl, and Houdret [15] went on to define a social contract as 'the entirety of explicit and implicit agreements between relevant societal *groups* and the sovereign (the government and any other actor in power), defining their rights and obligations toward each other' (p. 3). Bautista, in 2020, explored the notion of a social contract in health care developed from the economic and socio-legal lenses [13]. It was quite convenient to examine the current state of the *organisation*, PhilHealth, as being in the 'state of nature' or anarchy in the classical social contract or Hobbesian sense.

In relation to the organisation of an inclusive national health insurance scheme in a pluralistic health system, one may say that it is a source of conflict. It is, thus, also a source of measuring power relations among societal groups or the political economy view. Bloom, Standing, and Lloyd [16] covered the political economy perspective and examined the issue of power emanating from knowledge gaps in different health care social contracts. From an economic perspective, the conflict that arises from the access and exercise of the state's power over the public-private purse in health financing involves transaction costs. Transaction cost refers to the cost of bargaining, contracting, and monitoring [17]. Avoiding or minimising transaction costs underpins arguments, at both theory and policy levels, on the types of arrangements or governance systems to bring out societal or organizational outcomes. Mutuality lies in the consensus on the goals of efficiency, equity, and quality of care. Will the order established following the pandemic and the launch of the new UHC Act be one of breakdown or continuity?

From a conceptual point of view, a governance lens covers three alternative arrangements—markets, hierarchies, and networks (MHN). Hence, a transaction cost analysis can present the problem as an organisational and design issue. This framework has seen the wide application since the beginning of the new public management reforms in the 80s. It has informed changing managerial practice in health care in countries, particularly health systems similarly organised as the English National Health Service [18].

3.1 Market

This section investigates the nature of exchange or interactions in the health system. The starting point is considering interactions in health care or insurance as a transaction of exchange. The discussion on the features of health insurance, at the beginning of the chapter and from microeconomic theory, highlights the argument that health care and health insurance are unlike other commodities traded in the market. The nature of transactions in health insurance is such that premiums, or the price of insurance, and pay-outs, or claims, in the form of benefit services, are not equivalent to the price and quantity nexus in the normal demand (and supply) for goods [2]. Presently, under pandemic conditions, for instance, there is more certainty to the need for health insurance. However, insurance cover for a 'sure thing', given prevalence and transmissibility, will not be available, or when available will be quite costly. With uncertainty in the amount and timing of incomes, an inherent feature of informal work, health insurance may be unaffordable. If it is unaffordable, then there is a lack of effective demand (and supply is not interested in lower prices).

Willingness to pay for health insurance is between 1.18–1.39% of GDP per capita for a year's contribution from the 16 studies included in a systematic review [19]. The lack of a general understanding of the benefits of health insurance has been the point of entry for randomised controlled trials involving the informal sector in Vietnam, China, and Philippines [20–22]. Observations were made on whether those who were provided with more information on health insurance, its benefits, and how to access them in the country would behave differently from those that did not receive such information. Other tweaks to the field experiments included having transport vouchers and/or having some handholding navigators who directed and even accompanied study respondents to the insurance offices. Evidence gathered from these studies indicated small improvements in demand, but severe income constraints and the lack of affordability prevailed. Other reasons cited were related to the perception of poor quality of services covered and complicated enrolment procedures.

3.2 Hierarchy

In the original tenets of Coase [23], market transactions have zero transaction cost, and the decision to be in the hierarchical ordering, that is, establish the firm, is a way to counter increasing transaction costs [24]. Public policy applications highlight the costs to the hierarchical arrangements, that is, government institutions. The costs of government intervention can be assessed and compared to outcomes that would have risen had they been left to the market. The government's exercise of influence, if not control, on the behaviour of various agents, is a source of conflict. Balancing competing interests has its costs and benefits. In standard economics language, a

Pareto solution reconciles everyone's interests, with the winners compensating the losers. In the health system, a social contract solution holds when institutions come to an agreement or reconcile their interests for the common good, to achieve desired outcomes.

The government's role in the health sector, given the inherent failures in the market, is seen as being provider, funder, and regulator. Standard textbooks view regulations as correcting for market failures, particularly in sectors with high externalities, non-competitive markets, and with deep information asymmetries [25]. National health service types of systems, such as in the UK and Canada, started as largely state provision and funding. The late 80s to 90s saw their evolution into quasi-market organisations separating state provision from state funding. The provision remains with the state, but some institutions are governed by boards and can compete for state funds and across other state bodies [26, 27].

How the government succeeds in its role can determine its ability to manage conflict and establish order. From an economic organisation perspective, government mirrors vertical integration or the hierarchical structure. In a pluralistic economy, where the private sector is extensively involved, the government's ability to be a balancing force is affected by the extent to which providers and other groups influence the regulatory process. Government reaches to other agents to secure its goal of assuring and protecting the health of citizens. The capability of the government to enter into commitments, usually through contracts with other sectors, has a consequence for transaction costs in the interaction. Schuhmann and Bautista explored the nature of contracting envisioned in the new Philippine UHC Act [28]. Government regulators deal with its 'regulatory hands' through command and control, delegation to the professions to practice self-regulation, contracting, and/or through the use of incentives to elicit desired behaviour.

There is mixed evidence on the role of incentives in improving health service performance [29]. The use of incentives is attempt to counter the limitations of the regulatory approach in the light of 'influence activities' [30] or regulatory capture, leading to corruption and inefficient public services. Low powered incentives, such as low salaries, can impede actions towards creating greater efficiencies. It is in the compatibility of incentives with the goals set out that the directions of policy reforms and the preferences of the legislature and the bureaucracy can be discerned. Eijkenaar, et al systematic review of systematic reviews on the effects of pay-for-performance in health care did not find convincing evidence of cost-effectiveness and instead found persistent inequalities and some unintended consequences for unincentivized care [31].

Salazar [32] found shortcomings in financial reporting practices by PhilHealth, along with declining financial health from 2015. From 2006 to 2015, premiums exceeded benefit claims. Until 2013, premiums from paying members were the most important source of revenues. Average contributions from the informal sector payors were below premiums due, because of the overstatement in the members list and lack of tracking for delinquency in payments or inactive members. The category of non-paying members, those that received government subsidies widely instituted through the 'sin tax' law, grew by 37% in 2015. The study noted that 53% of benefit claims were made by non-paying members' benefits. Benefit claims from the informal economy were three times their premium contributions. The new UHC Act full implementation is expected to expand subsidies. Citing a study by Gertler and Solon [33] 86% of increases in funding to PhilHealth went to payments for health care providers as profits or higher salaries. Cross-subsidisation was maintained, with formal workers subsidizing benefits of other sectors on some periods, while subsidised members by government pro-poor programmes showed some volatility between negative and positive net contributions. The informal economy members were consistently at the receiving end of cross-subsidies. The medium-long term prospects of PhilHealth's net worth were not optimistic. In the midst of the fight against the pandemic, with the various anomalies in fund utilisation and employees' behaviour, the President of the country announced that he would make a request to Congress to abolish PhilHealth [34]. This remains an empty threat, however, as Presidential elections are scheduled for May 2022.

3.3 Networks

Referring to a 'broad set of collaborative approaches that are useful for bringing stakeholders together' [35], network arrangements can be considered a looser organisational form. Whether it can be viewed as a third-best alternative, when 'market fails' or 'regulations fail' is a normative question. A convenient view would be to see it as running along the same continuum—straddling the range of market and hierarchy, a hybrid of elements from both, plus other features. This is possibly an appropriate perspective for the subject of interest—the informal labour sector. This issue means balancing interests in informal sector's access to social health financing and health service benefits. To bring the interests of disadvantaged groups in the bargaining processes for the health care system's allocation calls for mediating institutions. The experience with financing cooperatives has not sustained membership for the individual economy programme. A leading cooperative planned to set up its own facility. The increased funding in the Z benefit programme (for catastrophic cases) and the coverage of some chronic disease maintenance costs, including dialysis, has seen private sector investments in stand-alone clinics. Patient groups have also been increasingly engaged in the discussion.

A review of widespread adaptation of networks in the British health service showed its growth among primary care, and other settings, and a reduction in the role of acute hospitals. The buzzword is 'collaboration' as opposed to 'competition' in market arrangements. It is also recognised in the participation of voluntary and private sectors in outsourced work 'commissioned' by the public sector. Performance tracking is a central activity. The latter's role has moved out from direct provision to one of purchaser or funder [36, 37].

From an LMIC perspective, collaboration takes place when the government reaches out to non-governmental organisations (NGOs) as well as the private sector to perform its traditional functions. The use of cooperative banks and other financial institutions to collect premium payments from the informal sector is one form. But it is not extensive enough to be called a network, rather public-private partnership has been used to describe it (Joint Learning Network). Examples remain few in the Philippines, surprisingly since it has one of the most vibrant NGO sectors actively engaging in the public sphere. There are no accounts of the private health clinic being contracted by the government to deliver primary care in geographically isolated areas where primary care needs abound. There are private clinics contracted to provide overseas employment medical checks, but for the most part, private and public health sectors in the Philippines are co-existing in parallel, if not in competition. Massive public sector investments in government health facilities have seen expanding capacities, in beds, laboratories, and services; while recent private sector developments have seen growing corporatisation and subsidiarity.

DOI: http://dx.doi.org/10.5772/intechopen.103720

Aside from income and basic demographic characteristics affecting demand for social health insurance from among the informal sector, trust in these institutions, from registering enrolment, collecting premiums, providing the medical services, including the attitudes of doctors and staff were found to determine willingness to pay and utilisation of services [38]. This was confirmed in a 2020 systematic review study by Miti et al. [39]. Willingness to pay for health insurance and pension scheme among informal economy sectors were strongly associated with income and trust. Experience of illness, attitude, and presence of doctors as well as distanced all played a role. The credibility of institutions to the people and trust are key to insurance products [40] and the lack thereof undermines it.

4. Social contract design elements to governance in the new UHC act

We explored insights into the relational arrangements to find an appropriate conceptual 'fit' for the tenets of governance under a social contract. The 'state of nature' in the current market and hierarchical provisioning is failing and heightens the need for alternative governance mechanisms. Will the new UHC Act establish order and be the disruption the Philippine health system needs? Universal health coverage in general and the Philippine UHC Act, in particular, represents a new agreement drawn by citizens' representatives and the government. This section discusses governance issues that impinge on UHC implementation and the operational trajectories affecting those in the informal economy. The intention of the section is not so much as a technical discussion, but to pinpoint directions for a re-thinking that needs to take place alongside post-pandemic reflections on the new normal.

4.1 Governance imperatives

At the centre of governance, analysis is transaction cost minimisation. The new settlement or social contract on universal health coverage poses the following boundary issues.

4.1.1 Primary institutions

The law divides the fiscal resources and responsibilities into two key agencies—the Department of Health (DOH) for population health and the PhilHealth for personal health. Local government units (LGUs), the owners of public health facilities, were given roles and tasks but hardly any authority and funding allocations. They received their own mandate through Executive Order 135 known as the Mandanas 'law' [41]. This order simply affirms the additional funding as part of their internal revenue allocation (from national taxes). Amounts will vary depending on the scale and scope of health services that are under them. The funding source for this is from the new tax sources recently introduced. The additional funds, however, are not earmarked for health. This constitutes one of the peculiarities of Philippine politics, 'giving a little for everyone'. LGUs will now confront the question whether paying premiums to PhilHealth for coverage of its 'nonpaying' constituents present a better deal for its resources as opposed to providing free services in their 'owned' facilities. The added resources strengthen the position of local units in bargaining with the health funders and bargaining costs incurred should be factored as part of transaction costs to the implementation of the new UHC Act.

4.1.2 Selective purchaser

The current dominant purchaser of health services is the Philippine Health Insurance Corporation. Managed as a quasi-government body or a government corporation, it has enjoyed some autonomy in its operations, with the Secretary of Health serving as Board Chairperson. The new UHC Act has provisions for reforms on board qualifications and membership, currently filled by government finance and health institutions, as well as private and labour sectors. PhilHealth's financial position has been under threat, and with providers faced with persistent payment delays (a case study was presented in ref. [13]), non-participation in the new UHC is also a threat by private providers [42]. Internally, implementation glitches and court cases against its officers and among themselves have dented the credibility of the institution. The President's threat of abolishing PhilHealth reverberates (as documented in [34]). The scale might be an issue, with the institution being a case of 'too big to fail'. Insights from the health insurance system in Thailand may point on the way forward, where the institutions are managed across three separate groups—civil servants, private employees, and the rest of the population [43]. Cross-subsidisation is valued for social solidarity purposes. However, in the Philippine case, scale economies are not realisable given human, technological, and systemic incapacities demonstrated by the organisation. The system before 1995 was tripartite as in Thailand when the Philippine population was 68.18 million and not 110.8 million as of 2021.

Failure to design and manage an information system accounts in large part for this failure, relying instead on manual authorisations and adjudication of claims. The system requirements are substantial and the treatment of information system costs as part of capital investment will bypass the 12% cap on administrative costs. However, government infrastructure projects in health care are known for being slow and cumbersome [44], requiring an inter-agency investment committee, among other concerns.

4.1.3 Provider and provider networks

Under the new UHC, every citizen will choose a General Practitioner (GP) for primary care, who will, in turn, be networked to diagnostic services and a tertiary hospital either at provincial or city levels. This introduces a novel element to the health system. Under the current system, anyone seeking care may go to any facility, doctor, or specialist so long as one is able to pay. Being tied to a GP entails availability or the supply of GPs in the first place. There is a viable public rural health system and stations spread across the archipelago. In more isolated and poorer areas, arrangements will need to be made for the outreach of public medical facilities or contracted private providers. In the towns and cities, private facilities will have to be willing to participate in the provider network to receive patients on referral. Participation will be on the application and submission of documentary requirements, including cost structure and subscription to the information system to be followed. This imposes costs to the private sector, as well as to local governments, the de-facto facility owners. Information technology (for example, telemedicine), including medical outreach, costs can be factored in for remote settings. Incentives are discussed in the UHC Act in the context of the private sector and LGU cooperation.

These governance options can inform whether the social contract embedded in the new UHC Act will minimise transaction costs and maximise benefits and health protection for the larger and more vulnerable groups. Mediating institutions and groups may be necessary to reach and navigate citizen engagement. The ability to contract would strengthen implementation efficiencies. When monitoring and delivery systems are not fully in place, leakages abound, responsibilities overlap, and absorptive capacities of both recipients and implementers are compromised. Implementation issues, gaps, and program weaknesses highlight the need for a more responsive approach when it comes to universal coverage of health insurance, particularly to the informal sector.

4.2 Other practicalities

Table 1 summarises the key concerns related to the health insurance coverage of the informal sector. This is not the place to be detailed as technical elements can be further studied. The table though captures the key elements of contributory schemes and how it relates to informal economy issues. It subsequently identifies strategic design and operating elements and how it can work out with UHC as the 'sweet spot' for the implementation of overall social protection programmes for the non-poor. The last column highlights what the system would be like if the schemes (social security, and health insurance) were to shift to and be under one platform of universal coverage.

There are high transaction costs involved in getting and maintaining participation of the informal sector. However, the new UHC Act considers everyone as a member. Even as their incomes and timing of receipt of incomes are not low enough to qualify them for national subsidies, transaction costs will be high trying to collect individually or tying individuals to a group. Localising subsidies from local tax sources will

Issues with the structure of health insurance schemes	Informal economy issues	Key operating or design elements	Universal coverage
Low coverage of the informal economy	Geographic location – reach and access to health facilities	Membership, enrolment become moot issues as new UHC mandates coverage for all	Reaching the population with information drives on rights and responsibilities and services
Intermittent contributions; drop-outs	Not too poor for pro-poor subsidies paid by the government from national taxes; no employer counterpart	Graduated subsidies from local government (LG) as part of business registration and renewals; Bundled with other contributions, for example, pension, accident insurance	No direct contributions from informal sector earning below a certain level (determined locally; with LG performance in the coverage of IFS tracked)
Utilisation of Health Care as part of benefits	High cost of care due to users' charges; Delayed care due to cost concerns Health insecurity due to nature of work	Member education Annual basic medical check-ups Assurance of adequacy in the supply of staff and medicines needed when on acute care for no balance billing arrangement	Inclusion in the No balance billing (NBB) arrangement Health technology assessment
Portability	Mobile population	Navigation and Information technology solutions	Information systems Use of Human Navigators Health passbook

Table 1.
Elements of schemes for the informal economy, design elements, and universal coverage.

bundle business registration with other businesses in the local city or municipality office, the usual point of entry for local business. This will encourage the informal economy to gain a foothold into formality with the enticement of free health insurance. Insuring the informal sector, based on the population discussed in section 2, and using the 10 year average and current PhilHealth premiums of P2,400, will amount to an estimated PhP51 billion (US$1 billion). This amount is approximately 5.1% of the annual health budget of the government. These subsidies will tie the funding of the informal economy health insurance coverage with the gains and benefits of coverage, not only as revenues (to fund local health facilities) but also as social capital, enhancing the credibility of local institutions [45].

Since local governments also 'own' the facilities, it is within their jurisdiction to provide free care for those in need, especially those that are not in the means-tested poor, of which many in the informal economy may fall under. No balance billing should be for all in the locally owned facilities and some capped charges, if outside the catchment area. Assurance of annual health checks will promote health maintenance and health security. The health technology assessment bureau, newly established under the UHC Act will recommend what the basic health service package will be.

Portability is key to universal health coverage. A Thailand study showed the popular use of non-designated facilities by low-income members [46]. Among mobile populations, working across provincial and city boundaries, where designated facilities may be accessed, local budget systems must be interconnected. Navigators or guides will be needed at facility levels. The Philippines' use of navigators has been singled out for promoting equity among the sponsored members [47]. Additionally, information systems that interconnect provider and patient information with the health insurance office and a health passbook, physical record on members' hands where utilisation and coverage in terms of fees are recorded, has been the glue to Taiwan's health insurance system, which began around the same time as PhilHealth in the mid-90s. Taiwavn achieved universal health coverage within the decade of its founding.

5. Conclusion

The study explored the issues related to the planning and inclusion of the informal labour sector into national health insurance schemes. While universal health coverage (UHC) may have raised this as a non-issue, with its coverage 'for all', resources flowing to the same structures for implementation will encounter the same problem of high transaction costs. A re-framing analysis that pushed the issue of transaction costs into the discussion showed that hierarchical or government structures wielding tight command and control are not informal sector—friendly. Informal sector participants may not fall within the strict proxy variable means tests for the poor. Thus, their non-inclusion in the no-balance-billing thrust of the UHC still creates high user charges which minimise the benefits of health insurance against any contribution on premiums they make.

The ability of the system to provide universal financial protection will still depend on subsidies managed through mediating institutions, including facilities, that need to be brought in as part of the new social contract. There will be widespread subsidies as the impetus for the universal health care Act itself is the anticipated fiscal space provided by the passing of new tax laws that included a tax on the sugar content of beverages. The pandemic has seen increased fiscal flows to the health sector; but more importantly, it surfaced the inefficiencies and corruption of the implementing agencies. The protection required in the new social contract is safeguarding the health insurance funds and the balancing of current expenditures and future funds sustainability. The rights and responsibilities implicitly pressed on citizens, providers, implementers by the new Act are directed towards ensuring the social insurance funds are protected. This is only possible if payments are made in terms of ability to pay, pay-outs designed based on needs, incomes drawn from the fund (by providers and other vendors) are fair, and systems and safeguards are in place for greater accountability. Universal health coverage is possible with better governance and undertaken in the spirit of a new social contract.

Acknowledgements

The article used parts of an unpublished report by the author submitted to the International Labour Organisation Regional Office in Bangkok, as part of a consultant's report on the project Stocktaking Study on Social Protection for the Informal Economy in 2018. Permission to recognise their copyright has been obtained and much appreciated.

Conflict of interest

No conflict of interest is declared by the author.

Author details

Maria Cristina G. Bautista
Ateneo de Manila University, Graduate School of Business, Makati City, Philippines

*Address all correspondence to: mcbautista@ateneo.edu

References

[1] Bitran R. Universal Health Coverage and the Challenge of Informal Employment: Lessons from Developing Countries [Internet]. Washington, DC: World Bank; 2014. [cited 2022 Feb 2] Available from: https://openknowledge.worldbank.org/handle/10986/18637

[2] Getzen T. Health Economics – Fundamentals and Flows. 2nd ed. Wiley; 2004, citing Arrow, K. Uncertainty and the welfare economics of medical care. The American Economic Review, 1963 (Volume 53, Number 5):941-973

[3] Bautista MC. Stocktaking study on social protection: needs and gaps for workers in informal employment in the Philippines. Thailand, Bangkok: Final Report Submitted to the International Labour Office; 2018. Citing: Department of Labour and Employment/ Philippines'Presentation at the South-South Knowledge sharing forum on Policy Innovations and Lessons Learned on Enterprise Formalisation to Achieve Decent Work in the Philippines through Peer-to-Peer Learning, 16-18 July 2018, Pasay City: Hotel Jen

[4] International Labour Organisation. Informality at a Glance: Snapshot by Countries: Asean and Other Countries in Asia and the Pacific. International Training Centre (ITC): ILO; 2017

[5] Kelly Bird CL. Philippines' COVID-19 Employment Challenge: Labor Market Programs to the Rescue [Internet]. Asian Development Bank; [cited 2022 Feb 1]. Available from: https://blogs.adb.org/blog/philippines-covid-19-employment-challenge-labor-market-programs-to-rescue

[6] Joint Learning Network for Universal Health Coverage. Closing the gap health coverage for non-poor informal-sector workers, 2015. Results for Development [Internet]. [cited 2022 Feb 2]. Available from: https://www.readkong.com/page/closing-the-gap-health-coverage-for-non-poor-417432

[7] Salvador D. Informal economy segmentation study: towards UHC in the Philippines – reaching and retaining members in the informal sector. Submitted to the Philippine Health Insurance Corporation by Alliance for Improved Health Outcomes (AIHO) and the Philippine Council for Health Research and Development, 2020

[8] Obermann K, Jowett M, Kwon S. The role of national health insurance for achieving UHC in the Philippines: A mixed methods analysis. Global health action. 2018

[9] Salazar DR. Financial condition and financial reporting of the Philippine Health Insurance Corporation, Philippine. Management Review. 2017. [cited 2022 Feb 2]; Available from: https://www.semanticscholar.org/paper/Financial-Condition-and-Financial-Reporting-of-the-salazar/f6c5a796879ce9f48ca179d40ce39e52a2670b22

[10] Rappler. 2021. SC affirms COA disallowance of P204M PhilHealth Benefits, 9 February. Available from: Rappler.com/nation/sc-affirms-coa-disallowance-of-philhealth-benefits/

[11] Capuno J, Kraft A, O'Donnell O. Filling potholes on the road to universal health coverage in the philippines. Health Systems & Reform. 2021;7(2):E1911473. DOI: 10.1080/23288604.2021.1911473

[12] Reyes MR, Santillan MC, Tacang AL, Vecina GS, Calabio DR, Tacang A, et al.

Field monitoring of the z benefits for breast cancer of the Philippine health insurance corporation. BMJ Open. 1 Aug 2015;5(Suppl 1). https://bmjopen.bmj.com/content/5/Suppl_1/bmjopen-2015-forum2015abstracts.9

[13] Bautista MC. The Philhealth case – Health care contracts and social contract in social health insurance. In: Schuhmann R, Eichhorn B, editors. Contractual Management. Berlin: Springer Vieweg; 2020. pp. 337-350. DOI: 10.1007/978-3-662-58482-8_11

[14] Williamson OE. Transaction cost economics: The natural progression. American Economic Review. 2010;**100**(3):673-690; citing Commons, J.R., 1932. "The problem of correlating law, economics, and ethics," Wisconsin Law Review, 8: 3-26

[15] Loewe M, Zintl T, Houdret A. The social contract as a tool of analysis: Introduction to the special issue on "framing the evolution of new social contracts in Middle Eastern and North African countries.". World Development. 2021 Sep;**1**(145):104982

[16] Bloom G, Standing H, Lloyd R. Markets, information asymmetry and health care: Towards new social contracts. Social Science & Medicine. 2008;**66**(10):2076-2087

[17] Williamson OE. The Economic Institutions of Capitalism: Firms, Markets, Relational Contracting. Vol. xiv. New York, London: The Free Press; 1985. p. 450

[18] Petsoulas C, Allen P, Hughes D, Vincent-Jones P, Roberts J. The use of standard contracts in the English National Health Service: A case study analysis. Social Science and Medicine. 2011;**73**(2):185-192

[19] Nosratnejad S, Rashidian A, Dror DM. Systematic Review of Willingness to Pay for Health Insurance in Low and Middle Income Countries [Internet]. Rochester, NY: Social Science Research Network; 2016. [cited 2022 Feb 2]. Report No.: ID 2804863. Available from: https://papers.ssrn.com/abstract=2804863

[20] Wagstaff A, Nguyen H, Dao H, Bales S. Encouraging health insurance for the informal sector: A cluster randomized experiment in Vietnam. Health Economics. 2016;**25**(6):663-674

[21] Barnighausen T et al. Willingness to pay for social health insurance among informal sector workers in Wuhan, China: A contingent valuation study. BMC Health Services Research. 2007, BioMed Central Open Access

[22] Capuno J et al. Effects of price, information, and transactions cost interventions to raise voluntary enrollment in a social health insurance scheme: A randomized experiment in the Philippines. Health Economics. 2010;**25**(6):650-662. DOI: 10.1002/hec.3291

[23] Coase RH. The nature of the firm. Economica. 1937;**4**(16):386-405

[24] Williamson OE. Transaction cost economics: The natural progression. The American Economic Review. 2010;**100**(3):673-690

[25] Will Bartlett HD, Roberts JA, Le Grand J. A revolution in social policy: Quasi-market reforms in the 1990s. Journal of Social Policy – J SOC POLICY. 1999;**28**:543-575

[26] Allen P. An economic analysis of the limits of market based reforms in the English NHS. BMC Health Services Research. 2013;**13**(1):S1

[27] Hood C. Public administration and public policy: Intellectual challenges for

the 1990s. Australian Journal of Public Administration. 2008;**48**:346-358

[28] Schuhmann R, Bautista MC. Contracting for health care under the new Philippine UHC Act. Vrue/WCL. 2021;**54**:98-115

[29] Macq J, Martiny P, Villalobos L, Solis A, Miranda J, Méndez HC, et al. Public purchasers contracting external primary care providers in Central America for better responsiveness, efficiency of health care and public governance: Issues and challenges. Health Policy. 2008

[30] Preker AS, Harding A, Girishankar N. Private participation in supporting the social contact in health: New insights from institutional economics. In: Recent Health Policy Innovations in Social Security. New York: Routledge; 2001. eBook ISBN: 9781351307444

[31] Eijkenaar J, Emmert M, Scheppach M, Schoffski O. Effects of pay for performance in health care: A systematic review of systematic reviews. Health Policy. 2013;**110**(2-3):115-130. DOI: 10.1016/j.healthpol.2013.01.008

[32] Salazar DR. Financial condition and financial reporting of the Philippine Health Insurance Corporation. Philippine Management Review. 2017. [cited 2022 Feb 2]; Available from: https://www.semanticscholar.org/paper/Financial-Condition-and-Financial-Reporting-of-the-Salazar/f6c5a796879ce9f48ca179d40ce39e52a2670b22

[33] Gertler P. and Solon, O. Who Benefits from Social Health Insurance in Developing Countries?, 2000. Available from: Researchgate.net/publication/228812916_WhoBenefits_from_Social_Health_Insurance_in-Developing_Countries

[34] Aguilar K. Duterte will ask Congress to abolish PhilHealth|Inquirer News [Internet]. INQUIRER.net. 2020 2020 [cited 2022 Feb 1]. Available from: https://newsinfo.inquirer.net/1341299

[35] Willis CD, Riley BL, Best A, Ongolo-Zogo P, Atkins, Borgatti, et al. Strengthening Health Systems Through Networks: The Need for Measurement and Feedback. 2022. Available from: https://core.ac.uk/display/282797991

[36] Ferlie E et al. Networks in Health Care: A Comparative Study of Their Management, Impact & Performance. University of Manchester; 2010. research.manchester.ac.uk/portal/en/publications/networks-in-health-care-

[37] ICF International. Evidence Scan: The Impact of Performance Targets Within the NHS and Internationally. Long Acre, London: Health Foundation; 2015

[38] Gilson L, Palmer N, Schneider H. Trust and health worker performance: Exploring a conceptual framework using South African evidence. Social Science and Medicine. 2005;**61**(7):1418-1429

[39] Miti J, Perkio M, Metteri A, Atkins S. Factors associated with willingness to pay for health insurance and pension scheme among informal economy workers in low-and middle-income countries: A systematic review. 2020. International Journal of Social Economics. © Emerald Publishing Limited 0306-8293; 2021;**48**(1):17-37. DOI: 10.1108/IJSE-03-2020-0165

[40] Banerjee AV, Duflo E. Poor Economics: A Radical Rethinking of the Way to Fight Global Poverty. PublicAffairs; 2012. p. 321

[41] World Bank. PHILIPPINES: Mandanas Ruling Provides Opportunities for Improving Service Delivery through Enhanced Decentralization [Internet]. Washington, DC: World Bank; 2022

Available from: https://www.worldbank.org/en/news/press-release/2021/06/10/philippines-mandanas-ruling-provides-opportunities-for-improving-service-delivery-through-enhanced-decentralization

[42] Crisostomo, S. Some hospitals to disengage from PhilHealth. |Philstar.com [Internet]. 2021. Available from: https://www.philstar.com/headlines/2021/11/02/2138349/some-hospitals-disengage-philhealth

[43] Tangcharoensathien V, Suphanchaimat R, Thammatacharee N, Patcharanarumol W. Thailand's universal health coverage scheme. Economic and Political Weekly. 2012;**47**(8):53-57

[44] Dayrit M, Lagrada L, Picazo O, Pons M, Villaverde M. The Philippines Health System Review. New Delhi: World Health Organization, Regional Office for SouthEast Asia. 2018;**8**(2)

[45] Watson J, Yazbeck A, Hartel L. Making health insurance prop-poor: Lessons from 20 developing countries. Health Systems and Reform. Taylor and Francis online. 2020;**7**(2). DOI: 10.1080/23288604.2021.1917092

[46] Paek SC, Meemon N, Wan TTH. Thailand's universal coverage scheme and its impact on health-seeking behavior. Springerplus. 2016;**5**(1):1952

[47] Capuno J, Kraft A, ODonnell O. Filling potholes on the road to universal health coverage in the Philippines. Health Systems and Reform. 2021;**7**(2):E1911473, DOI: 10.1080/23288604.2021.1911473

Chapter 5

An Assessment of the Effect National Health Insurance Scheme Capitation Payment to the Healthcare Facilities in Yobe State

Salisu Hassan

Abstract

With the transition of countries from financing healthcare through government revenue, general taxation, and out-of-pocket to Social Health Insurance in order to ensure the achievement of Universal Health coverage, the global health research community has made very important efforts to advance knowledge about the effects of various health schemes. Although there is a large amount of literature about the effects of various payment mechanisms, usually it does not focus on the effects of capitation payment to the healthcare facilities. To fill this knowledge gap, this study assessed the effects of National Insurance Scheme (NHIS) capitation payment on revenue generation, expenditures, utilization of funds, and enrollees' satisfaction with healthcare facilities in Yobe State, Nigeria. The framework of this study is system theory. The study employed a survey method to obtain both quantitative and qualitative data. Structured questionnaires were applied and key informant interviews were conducted. The study revealed that the capitation payment mechanism to the healthcare facilities impacted positively on the NHIS, providers, and the enrollees. Specifically, the study revealed that capitation increased the revenue of healthcare facilities, increased quality of services, improved provision of drugs and consumables as well as ameliorated the maintenance of infrastructures. Generally, capitation payment mechanism was found to increase competition between healthcare facilities and reduced the out-of-pocket expenses for healthcare by the enrollees. The study recommends proper monitoring and evaluation of the way capitation payments are made by the Health Maintenance Organizations to the healthcare providers. Also, National Health Insurance Scheme should ensure regular payment of capitation by HMO to facilities to avoid unnecessary delay of payment and finally, the capitation amount should be reviewed on regular basis by the National Health Insurance Scheme so that healthcare facilities would be funded adequately to provide qualitative services to the enrollees.

Keywords: capitation payment, healthcare facilities, health maintenance organizations, qualitative services

1. Introduction

The paradigm shift from financing healthcare through government revenue, general taxation, and out-of-pocket to social health insurance is not new. In most of the developing nations, reform on the purchasing side is moving hand in hand with development of pooling functions. According to Moreno-Serra and Wagstaff, many countries of Europe and Central Asia include case-based payment for tertiary care and capitation payment for primary care. Likewise, Nigeria has adopted a similar system of financing healthcare through these two major options of payment [1].

Since the flagged in the Formal Sector Social Health Insurance Programme in Nigeria in June, 2005 capitation payment has remained one of the social health insurance payment mechanisms to the healthcare facilities through the Health Maintenance Organizations (HMO).

Health Maintenance Organization is a private or public incorporated company registered by the National Health Insurance Scheme (NHIS) solely to ménage the provision of healthcare services through healthcare providers accredited by the NHIS [2]. HMO provides the following main functions:

i. effect timely payments to healthcare facilities;

ii. ensure the quality of healthcare services;

iii. ensure timely approval of referrals and undertake necessary follow up to complete referrals; and

iv. carry out continuous sensitization of enrollees [3].

In Nigeria, presently there are 94 registered HMOs that are responsible for the payment of primary, secondary, and tertiary health services to the healthcare facilities on behalf of NHIS. Primary healthcare services include: out-of patient care, immunization, surgical procedures, internal medicine, HIV/AIDS, obstetrics, gynecology, pediatrics, laboratory investigations, and emergency care [4]. These services are covered by capitation payment. All other procedures that cannot be handled at the primary level of care can be undertaken at the secondary level, which the HMO paid healthcare facilities as the fee for service.

Capitation is defined as a payment method where the provider is paid in advance, a predetermined fixed rate to provide a defined set of services for each individual enrolled with the provider for a fixed period [5]. Capitation usually occurs under Bismarck or social health insurance healthcare system [6]. Bismarck model involves people (those who need healthcare) paying a fee to a fund that in turn pays health care activities, that can be provided by state-owned institutions, other government body-owned institutions, or a private institution. It is different from the Beveridge system (or National Health Insurance Schemes) in which government or central authority takes the responsibility of collecting and pooling funds and also pays for providers [7].

Every year, the National Health Insurance Scheme (NHIS) in Nigeria has been paid a large amount of money in the form of capitation. In Yobe State alone from January to December 2021 approximately, NHIS paid about (USD$700985. 75) for the payment of capitation to the accredited healthcare facilities for primary services in the state [8].

If the amount of money in funds received as a capitation by the healthcare facilities is properly allocated by providers, then one may expect the following:

i. positive impact on the effective delivery of healthcare services to the enrollees,

ii. increase on providers' revenue and improvement in infrastructure of the healthcare facilities,

iii. enhance the welfare of the healthcare workers.

This study aims to test these hypotheses concerning the effect of capitation payment on healthcare providers in Yobe State. There is a large amount of empirical literature on the capitation payment method, which focuses on the nature of this payment mechanism, but in general, it does not address the potential effect of capitation on services provision, infrastructure, and other ways of efficient utilization of the capitation fund, nor are the challenges of capitation payment system described in Sub-Saharian African Countries. This study represents an effort to fill this gap in the literature using the experience of Yobe State of Nigeria, where capitation payment has been introduced within the National Health Insurance Scheme.

2. Theoretical framework

Our world is complex and made up of subsystems. These subsystems interact with each other and each has vividly coherent dynamics and defined boundaries. Ludwig von Bertalanffy developed the Systems Theory in 1932 with an aim of simplifying the world's complexity and making it more comprehensible to human beings. Basically, the theory aims at explaining how things function around us. The theory views the world as a set of smaller subsystems that humans utilize on a daily basis. For instance, a hospital is a system that has outputs, processes, and inputs. In itself, the National Health Insurance Scheme (NHIS) is part of a bigger health care system. This study is premised on System theory. NHIS as a system has many subsystems that contribute to its proper functioning. Therefore, NHIS must work hand in hand with the healthcare facilities, the enrollees, the Health Maintenance Organizations, the banks, the insurance companies, and the other stakeholders. Hence, the System theory is relevant to the present study and will be used to support our work. In this regard, NHIS gives inputs, which are the resources that are capitation to the healthcare facilities through the HMO, which they use banks to transact the fund to the facilities. When NHIS gives money to HMO for the payment of capitation to the healthcare facilities this is called the process. Therefore, when the healthcare facilities successfully received capitation funds from the HMO and utilize the fund for the purchasing of drugs, consumables, and the procurement of expenditures and give services to the enrollees this is called the output, which is the effect of capitation. This flow of money called capitation payment is represented in **Figure 1**.

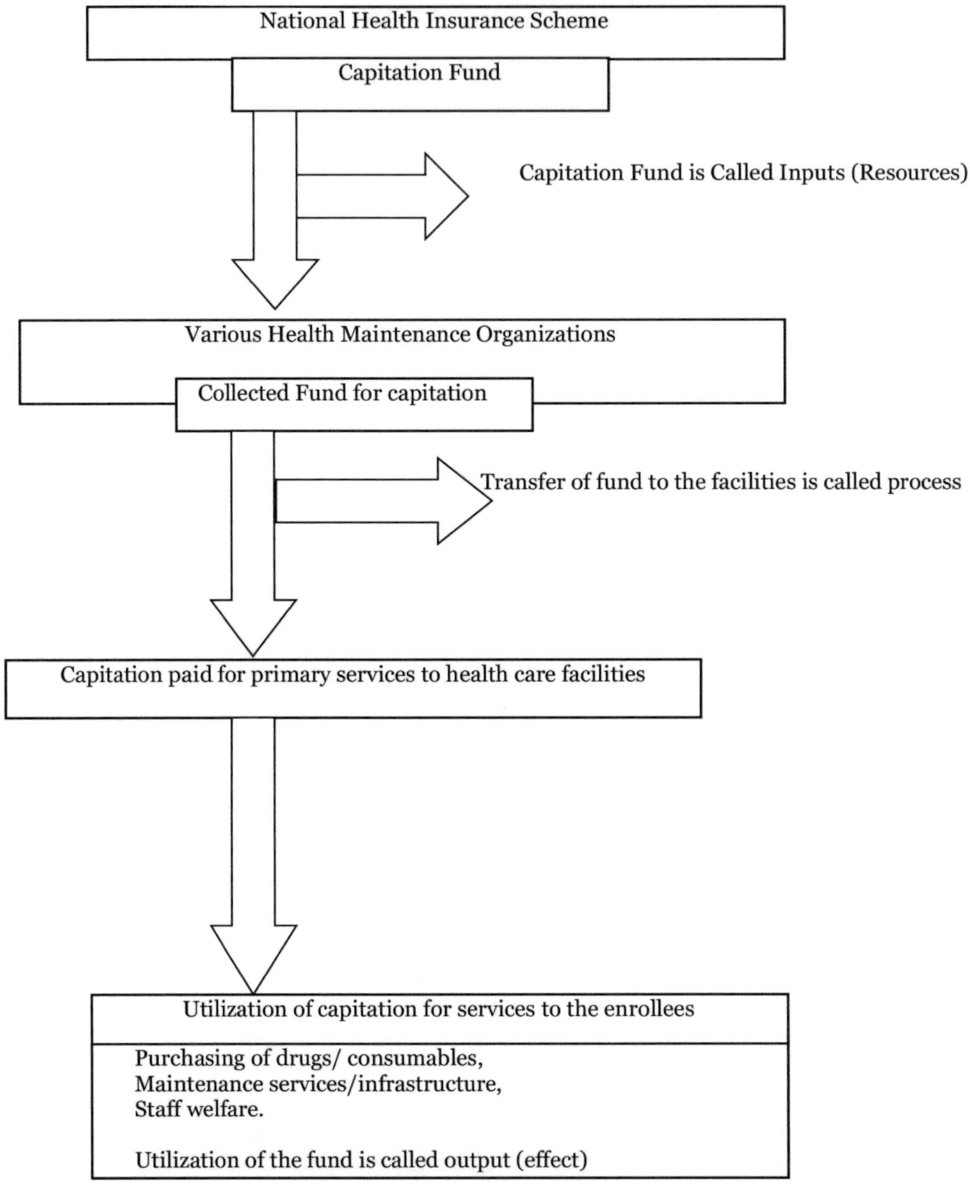

Figure 1.
How capitation payment is being made. Source: The Author, 2021.

3. Review on sub-Saharan Africa experiences

This subsection presents a brief review of the operation, outcomes, experiences, and perceptions of users and partners in the social health insurance scheme in Sub-Saharan Africa. The snapshot review on different experiences across several Sub-Saharan Africa is next summarized.

Barasa et al. examined the perceptions and experiences of informal sector people living in two of Kenya's provinces with contributory National Hospital Insurance Fund (NHIF). The study was qualitative in design, making use of data from carefully selected informants in the provinces. Findings revealed poor perception and experiences related to inadequate and inconsistent information about registration and membership process, affordability issues, and discrimination against NHIF patients over those paying out-of-pocket [9].

The governments in Africa often partner with private healthcare providers for better coverage of their health insurance schemes. Against this background, Sieverding et al. examined the perspective and experiences of private health providers with the National Health Insurance Scheme (NHIS) in Ghana and the NHIF in Kenya. The study was an interview-based survey with a qualitative research design. Interview responses were coded and content-analyzed thematically. Poor communication of requirements for registration/accreditation and complex accreditation process was reportedly the major constraint in Kenya in line with the finding of Barasata et al. [9]. The accreditation experience in Ghana differs as it was found to be mostly straightforward. Private healthcare providers participating in health insurance schemes reportedly perceived the schemes to be worthwhile but identified poor engagement due to poor communication as barriers to active participation in the scheme.

Against the backdrop of low enrolment level in health insurance schemes in Ghana, Duku et al. analyzed the differences in perceptions between the insured and uninsured of the non-technical quality of healthcare and a possible association between insurance status and perception of healthcare quality with a view to ascertain whether insurance status matters in the perception of healthcare quality or not. The study was a primary survey, using quantitative research design. Results show that those insured had a more negative perception of the scheme compared to the uninsured, indicating the quality of service received. This finding appears to corroborate the discrimination against patients insured under social health insurance over those paying out-of-pockets by Barasa et al. [10].

Fenny et al. comparatively examined access to social health insurance schemes in five sub-Saharan African countries including Ghana, Rwanda, Tanzania, Ethiopia, and Kenya with a special focus on access by the poor. Access is key to experience, and experience informs perception. In Rwanda, both the poor were observed to have comparable lower inequality access unlike Ethiopia and Ghana with large access inequality between the poor and the rich. Only about 2% of the poor in Ghana and Ethiopia reportedly had access to the social health program. Fraudulent claims, difficulty in identifying who are actually the poor, poor funding, policy inconsistency, and enrolling the poor into social health insurance schemes were identified as barriers to widespread access to the schemes [11].

Amu et al., performed a quantitative secondary study using demographic and health surveys data and; assessed variations in health insurance coverage in four African countries including: Ghana, Kenya, Nigeria, and Tanzania. The data were analyzed using bivariate and multivariate techniques. Findings revealed that coverage was highest in Ghana (Females =62.4%, Males =49.1%) and lowest in Nigeria (Females =1.1%, Males =3.1%). Age, level of education, residence, wealth status, and occupation were the socio-economic factors influencing variations in health insurance coverage in the countries [12].

Erlangga et al., examined the public health insurance impact on health care utilization, financial protection, and health status in low- and middle-income countries based on a systematic literature review. Findings revealed that the public health insurance schemes generally appear to increase healthcare utilization, offer appreciable financial protection to their users, and have a positive effect on the health of the insured [13].

Adeniran et al. investigated cesarean delivery (CD) experience among out-of-pocket (OOP) and health insurance clients in Ilorin, Nigeria with a special focus on pregnancy events and financial transactions for the CD. The study was quantitative in design, using randomized sampling and inferential statistics. Findings revealed that OOP payers are prone to catastrophic spending on health. The waiting time before reimbursement to healthcare providers was found to be significantly prolonged; private insurers reportedly offered earlier and higher reimbursement compared to public insurers. Suboptimal referral and transportation of health-insured clients were found [14].

Adewole et al., examined enrollees' knowledge about the National Health Insurance Scheme (NHIS) and satisfaction with health services provided under the scheme in a cross-sectional questionnaire-based descriptive study. Findings revealed that 67% of the respondents had good knowledge about the NHIS. Majority of the respondents reportedly paid for drugs, laboratory tests, consultation fees, and X-ray out-of-pocket (81.2%) to supplement their health insurance cover. Slightly more than half (52.8%) of the respondents were found to be satisfied with service delivery, under the scheme with female respondents being significantly more satisfied than their male counterparts [15].

The foregoing review shows that there is a mixed outcome, experience, and perspectives on the impact of health insurance scheme in Sub-Saharian Africa. A common experience across the countries captured in the review is discrimination against and/or exploitation of enrollees in the health insurance schemes compared to those who pay out-of-pocket. Communication barriers, bureaucratic delay in paying partnering private healthcare providers, and policy inconsistencies via politics appear to be central issues militating against effective service delivery and good experience of the schemes by enrollees. Coverage appears to be low in the subregion except for Rwanda's experience. Particularly in Nigeria, going by the reform in the National Health Insurance Scheme there is significant improvement in the coverage of the various segments of the population through the introduction of Group Individual and Family Social Health Insurance Program.

4. Methods

The survey design was used in this study. According to Kerlinger [16], a survey is the best research design for obtaining social facts, beliefs, and attitudes for both large and small populations to discover relative distribution and interrelation of sociological and psychological variables. Survey uses questionnaires, likewise, our study used questionnaires to obtain the data. Also, the survey has an interview, hence this study also uses key informant interviews to generate information to support data obtained from the questionnaire. In other words, this study employed a mixed research approach that is both quantitative and qualitative [16].

The quantitative data were obtained from the population of healthcare facilities' staff of 27 NHIS accredited hospitals and clinics in Yobe State. Convenient sampling was employed to select two officials in each of the healthcare facilities to make the selected 54 officials. Hence, 54 closed-ended questionnaires were distributed to the healthcare officials who are mostly the Medical Directors and the NHIS Desk Officers. Out of 54 questionnaires administered, 44 were successfully returned, which represents an 81.48% response rate.

The distributed questionnaires were used to gather data on the effect of capitation on revenue generation, efficient use of resources by the healthcare providers, and the data of whether the capitation payment is sustainable or not.

DOI: http://dx.doi.org/10.5772/intechopen.102545

Another questionnaire was used to obtain information regarding enrollee's satisfaction. This questionnaire instrument was administered to determine whether the enrollees were satisfied with the services of healthcare facilities or not. Prior to the distribution of this questionnaire, the sample size in this study was determined to be approximately 32,000 NHIS enrollees. By using a Survey Monkey sample size calculator, the sampling size arrived at 354 enrollees. Hence, 354 questionnaires were administered to the enrollees in the various healthcare facilities and the NHIS office of Yobe State. Out of the 354 administered questionnaires, 343 represent 96.89% response rate.

Moreover, qualitative data were obtained through the key informant interviews conducted with the 7 officials of the NHIS Yobe State Office.

The information obtained in these interviews was mainly used to support the quantitative data obtained from the questionnaires already administered. Also, the information regarding the challenges of the capitation payment system to healthcare facilities was obtained through key informant interviews.

For the data interpretation and analysis, descriptive statistics have been employed, that is to say, the data were presented using tables with frequencies and percentages. In the case of qualitative data, except on the information regarding the challenges of capitation payment, narrative statements of the key informant interview respondents' were directly presented to support or juxtapose the quantitative data that had already been presented.

5. Results

Table 1 shows the results obtained from the respondents to the question: "Does capitation increase the revenue of your healthcare facility?"

Table 1 presents data on whether the capitation payment to the healthcare facilities by the NHIS had increased the revenue of the facilities or not. Majority of the respondents 88.63% said the capitation paid by the NHIS through the Health Maintenance Organization (HMOs) had increased the revenue of the providers.

The view of the majority of the respondents who took part in this study was equally the view of the NHIS Coordinator Yobe State AlhajiDabo I. Abdullahi one of the key informants. He claimed that:

> *One of the objectives of the Scheme is to ensure the availability of funds to the healthcare sector for improved services. Without a doubt, the NHIS capitation payment to the healthcare providers has served as a fundamental way of generating the healthcare facilities' revenue. NHIS has been paying a lot of money for both public and private health care facilities [17].*
> *(KII with AlhajiDabo I. YobeState, NHIS Coordinator on, 4th November 2021)*

Table 2 shows the results obtained from the respondents to the question: "Do you efficiently utilize capitation resources in your healthcare facility?"

Table 2 sheds an insight on the effects of the utilization of the resources paid to healthcare facilities as a capitation by the Scheme. **Table 2** shows that the majority of the respondents 80.63% have agreed that the capitation paid to facilities have been used for the supply of drugs and other consumables.

More so, for the maintenance of the healthcare facilities, **Table 2** also shows that 56.81% of the respondents confirmed that the capitation has been utilized for the provision of infrastructure and other hospital equipment. Additionally, it shows that

Option	N	%
Yes	39	88.63
No	4	9.09
Not sure	1	2.27
Total	44	

Source: Field Survey, 2021. Note: N—number of respondents; %—percentage.

Table 1.
Effect of capitation in healthcare facilities revenue.

65.90% of the respondents proved that part of the capitation resources had been used for daily maintenance of the facilities.

In regards to the staff welfare, **Table 2** also shows that about 70.45% of the respondents have agreed that part of the capitation payment had been used for the improvement of the workers' welfare in the facilities.

The effect of capitation payment to the healthcare facilities in Yobe State is not only confirmed by the respondents in the table twos above but also the evidence below from the interview with the Yobe State Coordinator. The Coordinator Alh. Dabo I. Abdullahi commented like this:

> *The impacts of NHIS capitation payment to the healthcare facilities through Health Maintenance Organizations (HMOs) are tremendous. In my experience as Coordinator in the state, I came across many facilities that had judiciously utilized their capitation resources for purchasing qualitative drugs as well as facilitating infrastructural development in their facilities. However, in some facilities with a high number of enrollees, part of their capitation also had been utilized for the welfare of their staff [17].(KII with Alh. Dabo I. Abdullahi NHIS, Yobe State Coordinator, on the 4th November, 2021)*

Option		N	%
drug supply/consumables	Yes	39	88.63
	No	4	9.09
	Not sure	1	2. 27
Infrastructure/hospital equipment	Yes	25	56.81
	No	12	27.27
	Not sure	7	15.90
Maintenance and other services	Yes	29	65.90
	No	12	27.27
	Not sure	3	6.81
Staff welfare	Yes	31	70.45
	No	9	20.45
	Not sure	4	9.09
Maintenance and other services	Yes	29	65.90
	No	12	27.27
	Not sure	3	6.81

Source: Field Survey, 2021. Note: N—number of respondents; %—percentage.

Table 2.
Effect on efficient utilization of capitation resources by healthcare facilities.

Table 3 shows the results obtained from respondents to the question: "Do you think competition to have more enrollees increase among the healthcare facilities?".

Table 3 sheds light on how capitation payments by the NHIS to the healthcare facilities increase competition among the facilities in the state. About 79.54% of the respondents confirmed that capitation payment had increased competition to have more enrollees among the healthcare providers in Yobe State. This table indicates that, only 11.36% of the respondents said capitation did not increase competition.

The data were obtained from the key informant interview with Alh. Mansur Akilu, Head of Human Resources and Administration NHIS Yobe State reinforced the position of 79.54% of respondents in **Table 3**. The position is captured below:

> *I observed that the capitation system increased competition to acquire more enrollees. The private healthcare facilities are competing to provide quality services to their NHIS patients in order to have more people and to retain their existing customers. Undoubtedly, facilities with more enrollees get more money from capitation payments [18].*
> *(KII with Alh. Mansur Akilu, NHIS Head Human Resources and Admin Yobe State on 5th November 2021)*

Additionally, AdamuShuwa an Accountant in the Yobe State NHIS Office concur the above view where his opinion is expressed below:

> *Capitation payment had increased competition by the hospital to provide qualitative service with the view to have more customers. In Yobe State, sometimes the healthcare facilities stop collecting 10% co-payment on drugs in order to retain their enrollees and not change to other providers [19].*
> *(KII with AdamuShuwa, Accountant, NHIS Yobe State on the 5th November 2021).*

Table 4 shows the results obtained from the respondents to the question: "Do you satisfy with the services given to you by your chosen healthcare facility?"

Table 4 above presents the data on whether the enrollees are satisfied with the Scheme service or not. The table indicates that the majority of the respondents, about 72.23%, were satisfied with the Scheme services that have been given to them in their respective healthcare facilities. While 22.66% of the respondents that have taken part in this study said that they were not satisfied with the services given to them by the healthcare facilities.

Option	N	%
Yes	35	79.54
No	5	11.36
Not sure	4	9.09
Total	44	100

Source: Field Survey, 2021. Note: N—number of respondents; %—percentage.

Table 3.
Effect of capitation in the increase of competition among the facilities.

Option	N	%
Satisfied	255	77.23
Not satisfied	80	22.66
Not sure	8	5.09
Total	343	100

Source: Field Survey, 2021. Note: N—number of respondents; %—percentage.

Table 4.
Effect of capitation on the Enrollees' satisfaction.

One of the key informants Alhaji Abubakar Uthman, the Head of Quality Assurance, supports the view of the majority of respondents, about 72.23% that said they were satisfied with the services given to them. The key informant commented, thus:

> *NHIS is very serious about the quality of services given to its enrollees, hence, we are always engaging on the quality assurance visit to the healthcare providers. In Yobe State, knowing it by healthcare facilities, substandard service can lead to the finality on their side so they give services that would satisfy the enrollees [20]*
> *(KII with Alh. Abubakar Uthman SQA Yobe State, on 4th November 2021)*

Another view from Alh. Gambo Gwadabe of Enlightenment Division NHIS Yobe State on the enrollee satisfaction:

> *Enrollees usually come for a change of providers if they are not satisfied with the services given to them by the healthcare providers. NHIS gives the provision of change in order to make facilities to provide quality services to the customers.*

On top Alh. Gambo also stated the following:

> *Enrollees do not need only quality drugs or other services but also the cutesy, good reception, since from the gate of the hospital. Time is also crucial to the enrollees; customers are very happy with the provider that would promptly attend them without wasting much of their time [21].*
> *(KII with Alh. Gambo Gwadabe Head of Enlightenment NHIS, Yobe State on 6th November 2021)*

Finally, another key informant, Dr. Auwal Ibrahim expresses that:

> *Regular spot checks by the NHIS can boost the quality of services provided by the healthcare facilities, hence regular visits help NHIS to identify the lapses in healthcare facilities and recommend where to improve for better services to the enrollees [22].*
> *(KII with Dr. Auwal Ibrahim SQA NHIS Yobe State on 6th November 2021)*

Table 5 presented the data on whether the capitation payment would be sustained to the question and provides the answers "Do you think the capitation payment is sustainable?". Majority of the respondents, 77.27% confirmed that the capitation payment system is sustainable. Only 18.88% of the respondents that have taken part in this study said the system is not a sustainable kind of payment.

DOI: http://dx.doi.org/10.5772/intechopen.102545

Option	N	%
Yes	34	77.27
No	8	18.18
Not sure	2	4.54
Total	44	100

Source: Field Survey, 2021. Note: N—number of respondents; %—percentage.

Table 5.
Sustainability of the capitation system.

The qualitative data from the key informant interview referred to just below agrees that the capitation payment system would be sustainable. This view is the opinion of Alh. Sani Zakari of the Formal Sector Social Health Insurance Programme unit who stated, thus:

> *Since the flagging off of the formal sector program in 2005 capitation payment has continued to flourish as one of the best payments of the NHIS to healthcare facilities through the HMOs. In my own opinion capitation payment has come to stay.*
> *(KII with Sani Zakari Formal Sector, NHIS Yobe State on 4th November 2021)*

The findings of this study may be summarized as follows:

1. Capitation payment increases the revenue of the healthcare facilities in the state. About 83.63% of the respondents confirmed that capitation contributed to the revenue of HCFs in Yobe State;

2. Capitation has contributed to the efficient utilization of resources of the healthcare facilities in the state. Both qualitative and qualitative data of this study have shown that the majority of the respondents in the study have agreed on the fact that resources acquired from the capitation were used for the efficient supply of drugs/consumables, provision of infrastructures, maintenance of equipment as well as the improvement of the staff welfare;

3. Both the qualitative and quantitative data established that capitation has enhanced competition for acquiring more lives or enrollees by the healthcare facilities. Hence, this contributes to the provision of qualitative services to the enrollees;

4. The study seems to support the idea that capitation is one of the sustainable payment mechanisms of healthcare services by the NHIS. About 77% of the respondents believe that capitation is going to be sustained. As well almost all the key informant interviews agreed that capitation is a sustainable way of financing healthcare;

5. The study concludes that majority of the enrollees were satisfied with the services provided by the healthcare facilities in Yobe State;

6. The study infers that the capitation system may reduce the out pocket payment of healthcare services by the enrollees;

7. Finally, this study also gathers information about some challenges of capitation payment to the healthcare providers as the delay in payment by the HMOs, sharp practices by the HMOs, mismanagement of the fund by the healthcare facilities, default of making payment by the HMOs, and lack of monitoring of the utilization of the fund by the healthcare facilities.

As a result of the findings from key informant interviews, the following challenges of capitation payment to the healthcare facilities in Yobe State were created:

1. There is a delay of the capitation payment by the Health Maintenance Organizations (HMOs) to the healthcare facilities. Studies show that even though the NHIS gives money for the capitation to the HMOs, sometimes they refuse to transfer the money to the healthcare facilities in due time usually after every 3 months;

2. There are sharp practices and mismanagement of the capitation fund by some of the healthcare facilities;

3. There is inadequate monitoring of the way the capitation fund is used by the healthcare facilities.

6. Discussion

Evidence from both quantitative and qualitative data in this study has shown that capitation payment increases the revenue of the healthcare facilities. For instance, 88.63% of the respondents believed that capitation payments increased the revenue of the providers. In comparing the amount of capitation being paid by the National Health Insurance Scheme in Yobe State with that being paid by the Yobe State Contributory Healthcare Management Agency (YOTCHMA), NHIS pays more than the amount (YOTCHMA) pays per head to the healthcare facilities for the same kind of services. The National Health Insurance Scheme uses HMO as an intermediary for the payment of capitation, while the YOTCMA pays capitation directly to the healthcare providers.

However, capitation is not the only payment mechanism to the healthcare providers in Yobe State that is contributing to the revenue generation of healthcare facilities but also the fee for service. According to the NHIS [3], fee for service is payment made by HMO to secondary/tertiary healthcare providers that render service to enrollee, and can also be paid on a service basis for emergency cases.

Apart from fee for service, there is co-payment which also contributes to the revenue of healthcare providers. This is payment made by the enrollee to the accredited pharmacy provider at the point of service. It is 10% of the total cost of drugs dispensed per prescription in accordance with the NHIS Drugs price list [3].

Other forms of payment to providers include Per diem and co-insurance. The former is payment made by primary providers and HMO to secondary/tertiary healthcare providers for bed space (per day) during hospitalization, while the latter refers to the part payment made by the enrollee for treatment/investigation covered under partial exclusion list while the HMO pays the balance.

The findings of this study have shown that capitation payment to the health care facilities in Yobe State contributed to the efficient utilization of the facilities fund. Since the fund is coming prepaid before service is given to the enrollee, this would enable providers to budget for drugs and other consumables, adequately. Sometimes when the healthcare facilities have enough funds at their disposal, they are utilized for the purchasing of equipment and the maintenance of infrastructure, and the improvement of staff welfare. This view was confirmed by the quantitative data in **Table 2**, for instance, where a majority of the respondents 88.63% have agreed that providers used the part of the capitation money paid to them for the purchase of drugs and consumables.

When comparing the utilization of funds generated by the healthcare facilities from capitation payment and other payment mechanisms such as fee for service usually, the generated fund from capitation is used for the procurement of drugs and consumables. Fund from fee for service payment usually comes after service is provided to the enrollee and it takes time to be collected from the HMO on behalf of NHIS. There are various protocols before the fee for service fund is being delivered to the healthcare facilities. Before accessing the fee for service payment from the HMO, a provider must request for referral code and after providing services the provider must send a claim to the HMO before payment would take place. According to National Health Insurance Operational guidelines of (2012) when the provider is unable to send a claim within 3 months of given service to the enrollee, that payment would not be paid.

This study confirmed that the capitation payment mechanism contributed to the increase of competition among the healthcare providers in Yobe State. In **Table 3** of this study, 79.54% of the respondents believed that capitation payment to healthcare facilities increases competition. In Yobe State, there are some healthcare facilities that are competing in terms of quality of care in order to have more enrollees so that more money can be received from capitation payment. According to an unpublished NHIS report (2021), some healthcare facilities are not collecting 10% copayment of drugs in order to attract more enrollees and retain the existing ones not to change to other facilities.

Concerning customers' satisfaction, the result of this study presented in **Table 4** points to the trend of satisfaction. Indeed, the majority of the NHIS enrollees in Yobe State were satisfied with the services provided. This may be explained by the way healthcare facilities are treating people in order to retain them in their facilities so that they would not change to other ones.

Regarding capitation payment sustainability, the majority of the respondents, about 78% in this study confirmed that the payment system should be continued and sustained, perhaps because of the positive impact of the payment method on the healthcare facilities. According to the unpublished report from NHIS (2021), since the flagging off of the Formal Sector Social Health Insurance Scheme, capitation payment mechanisms have been used for the payments of primary healthcare service in the whole federation, which may sign the potential sustainability of this payment method.

Without a doubt, capitation serves as a critical source of income to the healthcare facilities. It also promotes adherence to guidelines and policies and encourages providers to work better and give health education to patients. However, in this study, some challenges associated with the capitation payment mechanism were identified, which need to be addressed by the National Health Insurance Scheme so that qualitative services will continuously be provided by the accredited healthcare facilities in the Yobe State.

7. Conclusion

This study proved the capitation payment system in social health insurance financing positively impacted the Scheme, in the healthcare facilities availability, and the health of enrollees themselves. This study also showed that capitation had increased the revenue of the healthcare facilities in Yobe state. The findings obtained here suggest that the fund generated by capitation is mainly used to pay for the provision of drugs, consumables, and the infrastructural development. Capitation payment appears to have improved competition among the healthcare facilities for enrollees and to retain the existing ones. Moreover, capitation seems to reduce out-of-pocket healthcare expenses of the enrollees in Yobe state. Finally, despite limitations, the present study provides an overall framework that can be utilized to guide future research and data collection efforts for evaluating the result of capitation payment not only in Yobe State but in the country at large.

Based on the findings of this study, the following recommendations are provided to the National Health Insurance Scheme:

1. The Scheme should engage in proper monitoring and evaluation to the healthcare facilities to know the level of the compliance on how the capitation funds are being utilized;

2. The Scheme should put more effective measures to ensure that the HMOs are transferring the capitation payment promptly without delay. That is to ensure effective reconciliation of the fund given to the HMOs and the healthcare facilities;

3. The capitation amount should be reviewed from time to time by the NHIS so that healthcare facilities would be funded adequately to provide qualitative services to the enrollees.

4. According to the theoretical framework used in this study, the National Health Insurance Scheme is a system, therefore, in order to be more successful, there is the need to integrate all its subsystems together that are the stakeholders. A good provider payment method has to address and be implemented within strong support systems. Wider systems issues of importance in developing and implementing a successful provider payment method include governance and accountability, financial management and stakeholder relationships, management information systems, monitoring, and evaluation.

Acknowledgements

First and foremost, my gratitude goes to Ana Cink Author Service Manager IntechOpen Limited, and Professor Aida Isabel Tavares for their encouraging me to write a chapter in this book. I also appreciate all the staff of the National Health Insurance Scheme, Yobe State Office, Nigeria for their support toward the success of this writeup. I also use this medium to thank Alh. AbdulsalamBala of Ama consulting for encouragement to me. Last but not the least, I am grateful to Dr. Emmanuel Jegede of the Department of Theater and Performing Arts Ahmadu Bello University Zaria, Nigeria for his advice to ensure the success of this work.

A. Appendix

APPENDIX I

RESEARCH CONSENT FORM

The researcher is conducting an interview for the purpose of gathering information regarding the topic "An Assessment of the Effect of National Health Insurance Scheme capitation payment to the Healthcare Facilities in Yobe State".

The information gathered from this study is going to be used for producing a Chapter in a Book tittle "Health Insurance" which is to be edited by Professor, Aida Isabel Taveres which would be published by IntechOpen, London. Your response will be treated with confidentiality and for the purpose of the study only.

Please, by filling your name and signature it means that you have accepted the following conditions:

I confirm that I have read the purpose of this study and also:

1. I Agree to take part in this interview
2. I agree to the use of my quotes and
3. I agree to use my name for the purpose of this publication.

Name of the Participant	Date	Sign
Alh. Dabo I. Abdullahi State Coordinator	4/11/2021	
Alh. ABUBAKAR USMAN SQA	4th NOV. 2021	
Adamu Muhammed Shuwa Actts	5th/11/2021	
Alh. Gambo Gwadabe Enlightment	6th/11/2021	
Alh. SANI ZAKARI FORMAL SECTOR	6th/11/2021	
AWWAL IBRAHIM SQA	6th NOV, 2021	
Alh. MANSUR AKILU Human/R	6th NOV, 2021	

Name of the Researcher
HASSAN. Salisu, Ph.D — 10th November, 2021

B. Key informant interview guides for the staff of national health insurance scheme Yobe State office

The researcher is conducting a study on the topic "An Assessment of the Effect of National Health Insurance Scheme capitation payment to the Healthcare Facilities in Yobe State". The study is for the purpose of producing a chapter in a book titled "Health Insurance" which is to be edited by Professor Aida Isabel Tavares and to be published by IntechOpen.

Name of the Respondent ——————————————.
Department——————————————

The following are the expected questions for the interview, please for your preparation.

1. What do you think are the ways in which Healthcare Facilities in Yobe state utilize their capitation fund under the Formal Sector Health Insurance Programme?

2. What is your opinion about the quality of services given to the enrollees by the Yobe State Healthcare Facilities?

3. Do you think enrollees are satisfied with the services given to them by Healthcare Facilities in this State?

4. Do you think the capitation payment is sustainable?

5. What do you think are the challenges of capitation payment system?

6. Please what are the possible solutions to the challenges of the capitation payment system to the Healthcare Facilities in Yobe State?

Thank you for your responses.
Hassan Salisu Ph.D.

C. Study questionnaire for the representatives of health care facilities

The researcher is conducting a study on the topic "An Assessment of the Effect of Capitation Payment to the Healthcare Facilities in Yobe State". The study is for the purpose of producing a chapter in a book titled "Health Insurance" which is to be edited by Professor Aida Isabel Tavares and to be published by IntechOpen. Please we need your maximum cooperation and your response will be treated with confidentiality and for the purpose of this study only.

Type of Healthcare Facility ——————————————————
Rank/Position of the Healthcare Facility's representative——————————

Questions

S/N	Questions	Responses		
		Yes	No	Not sure
1.	Does capitation increase the revenue of your healthcare facilities?			
2.	Do you use fund generated from capitation to buy drugs/consumables for the NHIS enrollees?			
3.	Do you use the fund generated from capitation to build infrastructures or purchase hospital equipment?			
4.	Do you use fund generated from capitation for the provision of staff welfare?			
5.	Do you use the fund generated from capitation for maintenance and other services in your facility?			
6.	Do you think as a result of capitation payment healthcare facilities compete to have more enrollees?			
7.	Do you think capitation payment mechanism to the healthcare facilities would be sustained?			

Thank you for your response.
Hassan Salisu, Ph.D.

D. Questionnaires for the national health insurance scheme enrollees'

The researcher is conducting a study on the topic "An Assessment of the Effect of National Health Insurance Scheme capitation payment to the Healthcare Facilities in Yobe State". The study is for the purpose of producing a chapter in a book titled "Health Insurance" which is to be edited by Professor Aida Isabel Taveres and to be published by IntechOpen. Please we need your maximum cooperation and your response will be treated with confidentiality and only for the purpose of this study.

Organization ——————————————————
Your Healthcare Facility ——————————————————

Please tick the appropriate box.
Question: do you satisfy with the services given to you by your chosen Healthcare Facility?
Yes ☐
No ☐
Not sure ☐

Thank you for your response.
Hassan Salisu, Ph.D.

Author details

Salisu Hassan
National Health Insurance Scheme, Programmes Department, Yobe State, Nigeria

*Address all correspondence to: salisu2015.sh@gmail.com

References

[1] Moreno-Serra, Wagstaff. System wide impacts of hospital payment reforms: Evidence from Central and Eastern Europe and Central Asia. Journal of Health Economics. 2010;**29**(2010): 585-602

[2] National Health Insurance Scheme. Operational Guidelines. Abuja: Corporate Headquarters; 2005. p. 45

[3] National Health Insurance Scheme. Operational Guidelines. revised ed. Abuja: Corporate Headquarters; 2012. p. 4

[4] National Health Insurance Scheme. Benefit Package and Drug Lists. Abuja: Yalliam Press Ltd, P14 Headquarters; 2021

[5] Langenbrunner, Cashin and O' Dougherty. Designing and Implementing Healthcare Provider Payment Systems. World Bank Group, Washington. DC. 2010. Available from: https://openknowledge.worlbank.org/handle/10986/13806

[6] Hoctor T. 11 Beveridge or Bismarck? Choosing the Nordic model in British healthcare policy 1997–c. 2015. In: The Making and Circulation of Nordic Models, Ideas and Images. Vol. 209. London: Informa UK Limited; 2021

[7] Moisidou A. Beveridge, Bismarck and Southern European Health Care Systems: Can we decide which is the best in EU-15? A statistical analysis. European Journal of Natural Sciences and Medicine. 2019;**2**(1):28-35

[8] National Health Insurance Scheme. Enrollee Register, January to December, 2021. Abuja: Corporate Headquarters; 2021

[9] Barasa EW, Mwaura N, Rogo K, Andrawes L. Extending voluntary health insurance to the informal sector: Experiences and expectations of the informal sector in Kenya. Wellcome Open Research. 2017;**2**:94. DOI: 10.12688/wellcomeopenres.12656.1

[10] Duku SKO, Nketiah-Amponsah E, Janssens W, Pradhan M. Perceptions of healthcare quality in Ghana: Does health insurance status matter? Amsterdam Institute of Global Health Development, Amsterdam, Netherlands. PLOS ONE. 2018;**13**(1):e0190911. DOI: 10.1371/journal.pone.0190911

[11] Fenny AP, Yates R, Thompson R. Social health insurance schemes in Africa leave out the poor. International Health. 2018;**10**(1):1-3. DOI: 10.1093/inthealth/ihx046

[12] Amu H, Dickson KS, Kumi-Kyereme A, Darteh EKM. Understanding variations in health insurance coverage in Ghana, Kenya, Nigeria, and Tanzania: Evidence from demographic and health surveys. PLOS ONE. 2018;**13**(8):e0201833. DOI: 10.1371/journal.pone.0201833

[13] Erlangga D, Suhrcke M, Ali S, Bloor K. The impact of public health insurance on health care utilisation, financial protection and health status in low- and middle-income countries: A systematic review. PLOS ONE. 2019;**14**(8):e0219731. DOI: 10.1371/journal.pone.0219731

[14] Adeniran A, Aun I, Fawole A, Aboyeji A. Comparative analysis of caesarean delivery among out-of-pocket and health insurance clients in Ilorin, Nigeria. Nigerian Postgraduate Medical Journal. 2020;**27**(2):108-114. DOI: 10.4103/npmj.npmj_181_19

[15] Adewole DA, Adeniji FIP, Adegbrioye SE, Dania OM, Ilori T.

Enrollees' knowledge and satisfaction with National Health Insurance Scheme Service Delivery in a Tertiary Hospital, South West Nigeria. Nigerian Medical Journal: Journal of the Nigeria Medical Association. 2020;**61**(1):27-31. DOI: 10.4103/nmj.NMJ_126_18

[16] Kerlinger FN. Foundation of Behavioural Research. 3rd ed. New York: Holt and Winston Inc; 1973. p. 119

[17] Abdullahi DI. NHIS Yobe State Coordinator on "An Assessment of the Effect of National Health Insurance Scheme Capitation payment to Health Care Facilities in Yobe State". 2021

[18] Akilu M. NHIS on "An Assessment of the Effect of the NHIS Capitation Payment to the Healthcare Facilities in Yobe State". 2021

[19] Shuwa A. NHIS Yobe State on "An Assessment of the Effect of the NHIS Capitation Payment to the Healthcare Facilities in Yobe State". 2021

[20] Uthman A. SQA, NHIS Yobe State on "An Assessment of the Effect of NHIS Capitation Payment to the Healthcare Facilities in Yobe State". 2021

[21] Gwadabe G. Enlightenment NHIS, on "An Assessment of the Effect of NHIS Capitation Payment to the Healthcare facilities in Yobe State". 2021

[22] Auwal I. SQA NHIS on "An Assessment of the Effect of National Health Insurance Scheme Capitation Payment to Health Care Facilities in Yobe State". 2021

Section 3

Health Insurance in High Income Countries

Chapter 6

Complementary Health Insurance in Slovenia

Tit Albreht, Marjeta Kuhar and Valentina Prevolnik Rupel

Abstract

Almost all health care services in the Slovenian basic benefits package are paid for from two financial sources: compulsory and complementary health insurance (CHI). Although this is unusual, around 90% of the population is insured under CHI. CHI covers the costs of copayments for most of the services. One of the advantages of the CHI is that it enables the public sector to shift the costs of service onto the private sector, which can compensate for the higher costs through premiums. Its administrative costs are low, the risk selection is low due to the equalisation schemes in place, and costs of copayments for the socially weak are covered by the state budget. Out-of-pocket costs are low due to most of the population being insured in CHI. On the other hand, there are many disadvantages of this unique amphibian health system. Besides the higher complexity and costs of such a health insurance system, CHI premiums are flat and regressive. The voluntary nature of CHI is highly questionable as the copayments can be as high as 90% of the total service costs. And last, but not least, CHI removes an incentive for the providers and payer to aim for efficient services.

Keywords: complementary health insurance, Slovenia, risk selection, inequality, efficiency

1. Introduction

Slovenia is usually counted among the countries whose health care financing system is Bismarckian. However, the Slovenian health care financing system is »biseridging« and getting more and more mixed. Most of the elements that are typical for a pure Bismarckian system, namely association of rights with labor status and no government interference, are not present anymore and lots of innovative elements entered the health care insurance space in the last decades.

Relatively, the Slovenian health care system ranks well across many indicators. Life expectancy has increased in the last two decades and is equal to the EU average of 80.6 years. Health spending is lower than the EU average (US$ PPP 2283 in 2019), and from the viewpoint of the benefits package, the accessibility to health services is almost universal. Due to its complementary health insurance and universal coverage, the financial protection is high-the out-of-pocket expenditures are one of the

IntechOpen

lowest in the EU, catastrophic spending is low, and unmet needs due to costs are low. The mounting problem is long waiting lists for specialist care and lack of health care personnel, especially in primary care [1].

In the following subchapter, we will describe the basic features of the health insurance system in Slovenia but will mostly focus on the concept of complementary health insurance and its role in the Slovenian health care system. On one hand, the institution of complementary health insurance brought Slovenia in front of the Court of Justice in Luxembourg; on the other hand, it played a crucial role in the economic protection of Slovenian citizens through the economic crisis between the years 2008 and 2013. Saying that it is necessary to point out that many adjustments have been introduced to complementary health insurance to ensure equal conditions for inclusion into the scheme for all citizens regardless of their age and gender and to ensure equal accessibility to complementary health insurance for all citizens is guaranteed without risk selection. In spite of all the adjustments, the nature of complementary health insurance is still ambiguous-it is declared voluntary but is in fact compulsory. Furthermore, it is run by private insurance companies while its package of services is completely dependent on the definition of services covered by compulsory health insurance does put the private providers into a subordinate position.

2. Health insurance system in Slovenia

According to the last available data, the public expenditures for health care in Slovenia amounted to 72.8% of THE (total health expenditures) in 2019, 69.4% being compulsory health insurance and 3.4% government expenditures. The private expenditures for health care amounted to the remaining 27.2%, from which 11.7% are out-of-pocket expenditures and the rest (15.5% of THE) are voluntary insurance schemes. The Health Care and Health Insurance Act (1992) defines more types of voluntary health insurance in Slovenia, which are as follows:

1. Complementary health insurance, which covers the difference between total price of the service and share of the price of this service covered by compulsory health insurance. This difference is in case of no complementary health insurance covered in a form of copayments.

2. Substitutive health insurance, which substitutes the coverage for services (and not more) that would otherwise be covered by the compulsory health insurance, including copayments. It is intended for persons that according to the legislation cannot be insured in the compulsory health insurance scheme. As substitutive health insurance is intended for specific population groups only that might for some reason be excluded from the compulsory health insurance – legislation in Slovenia does exclude any specific population groups, such as high-earners – therefore this type of insurance is not available.

3. Supplementary health insurance that covers costs of health care services that are not covered by compulsory health insurance, complementary health insurance or substitutive health insurance. They cover faster access to services or increased consumer choice.

4. Parallel health insurance is insurance for services that are covered by compulsory health insurance but are realized following different procedures and different conditions.

All persons who have a permanent residence in Slovenia must have compulsory health insurance in Slovenia. At the end of 2021, there were 3214 (0.15%) uninsured persons with permanent residence. Mostly, these are persons whose status is undergoing change, for example, students who finished their studies and are getting employed.

Compulsory health contributions are the largest source of income in the Slovenian health care system. Contribution rates, which are employment-based and paid from gross income, vary by group and type of employment of insured individuals. Employees pay 6.36% of their gross income, while employers pay 6.56% for illness and injury out of work plus an additional 0.53% for injuries at work and occupational diseases. The total contribution rate hence amounts to 13.45% of gross income. The contribution rates are the same for self-employed, though their contribution base is equal to the gross pension base and cannot be lower than 60% of the last-known average annual wage [2]. The contributions for the unemployed are covered by National Institute for Employment; the contributions for the pensioners are covered by Pension and Disability Insurance Institute at a 5.96% contribution rate from net pensions.

The Health Care and Health Insurance Act (1992) defines the rights to health care alongside their coverage within compulsory health insurance. The coverage ranges between 10% and 100%, depending on the services. A minimum of 90% of the cost of services is covered for organ transplantation and urgent surgeries, treatment abroad, intensive therapy, radiotherapy, dialysis, and other urgent interventions included in the basic benefits package; 80% of the cost of treatment for reduced fertility, artificial insemination, sterilisation, and abortion; specialist surgery; nonmedical care and spa treatment in continuation of hospital treatment with the exception of non-occupational injuries; dental care and orthodontics; orthopedics; hearing and other aids and appliances; 70% of the cost of medications from the positive list and for specialist, hospital and spa treatment of non–work-related injuries.

A maximum of 60% is covered for non-emergency ambulance transportation, medical and spa treatment; 50% of the cost of ophthalmological devices and adult orthodontic treatment; 25% of the cost of pharmaceuticals from the intermediate list.

The remaining shares of the services must be covered by out-of-pocket copayments. As these can reach quite high levels, 95% of the population, liable to purchase the coinsurance, is insured with complementary health insurance. Due to the high share of the population covered, complementary health insurance is by far the main type of voluntary health insurance in Slovenia and has been described as 'compulsory' or 'de facto essential' [3].

There are three companies that offer complementary health insurance in Slovenia: Vzajemna, Generali, and Triglav zdravje. The premium is a flat rate and equal for everyone. The monthly premium amounted to an average of 34 EUR in 2021.

To ensure that the companies do not offer coverage only to low-risk or healthy and young individuals, the Ministry of Health (MoH) introduced the risk-equalisation scheme in 2005. According to the scheme, contributions are reallocated among the insurance companies based on the age and gender of the insured. The aim is to equalize the portfolio structures (according to the age and gender) of the insurance companies. The funds are transferred from insurance companies with more favorable risk portfolios to insurance companies with less favorable portfolios, the intention being the equalisation of differences in risk structures.

Individuals who have taken out supplementary health insurance pay premiums to the insurance companies, who in turn pay the full costs directly to the respective health care provider. As the basic benefit package in the compulsory scheme comprises a wide range of services, there is little room for supplementary health insurance. Parallel insurance, which covers services such as faster access to medical treatment, nonmedical services in hospitals, and higher-quality materials, with providers already offering services within compulsory health insurance, gains in popularity. Since 2017, the share of other voluntary health insurance (VHI) policies has been increasing, mostly due to ever-lengthening waiting lists in the public health care system. In 2019, supplementary and parallel insurance was purchased by 26% of the population (2011: 5.6%; 2015: 18.9%); however, their premiums still represent a small share (4.55%) of all voluntary health insurance premiums.

3. Financial and coverage overview

In 2018, public expenditure on healthcare in Slovenia amounted to 5.8% of GDP (gross domestic product) [4]. Over the last 10 years (**Figure 1**), the evolution of public expenditure on health reflects the fluctuations related to the adoption of certain measures and the economic cycle, but during this whole period, it remained at around 6% of GDP. The same is true for total current health expenditure, which reached 7.9% of GDP in 2018, the lowest level in the last 9 years, which is also below the EU average of 8.4 % of GDP [1, 4, 5]. Existing policies have been successful in maintaining spending levels, but there have been problems with the financial performance of public health facilities, and waiting times have increased, worsening the accessibility of health services [1, 5].

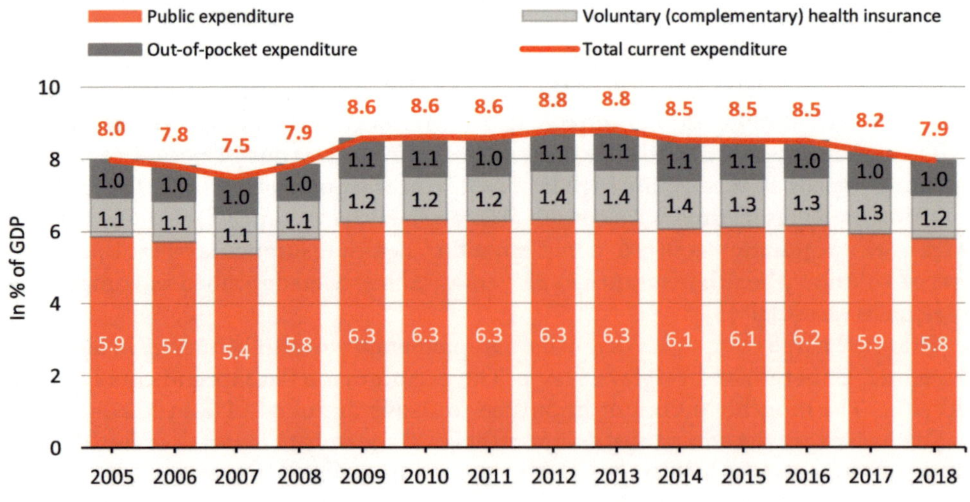

Figure 1.
Health expenditure by financing scheme, in % of GDP, 2005–2018. Source: Institute for Macroeconomic Analysis and Development, 2019 [5].

Expenditure on VHI amounted to 1.2% of GDP in 2018, while it increased by about 0.1–0.3% of GDP between 2009 and 2018. Total health expenditure by functions and sources of funding in Slovenia (2006-2019) is shown in **Figure 2**. Complementary health insurance is an additional source of funding for the health system, as much as 95% of the population is enrolled. According to the Health Care and Health Insurance Act (Article 23), most health services involve high copayments for most of the population. Only certain diseases, children, and young people under 26 years of age enrolled in school are fully covered by compulsory health insurance. The risk of copayments is hence very high [1].

Since 1992, the share of copayments has gradually increased due to a lack of public funding, especially during the last economic crisis. The income-independent single premium is the largest weakness of complementary health insurance in the system. This means that the system is regressive, although it should be supported by income solidarity given the high risk of copayments. In 2016, for example, the annual premium was equivalent to 62% of the net monthly minimum wage, 33% of the average net wage, and 57% of the average net pension [4, 6]. The regressive nature of this source was significantly reduced in 2012 when new social legislation introduced the automatic transfer of user fees from the state budget for welfare recipients. This benefit had already been introduced in 2009, but until 2012, it was not automatically linked to eligibility for social assistance [1].

Almost every permanent resident of Slovenia is entitled to the health benefits covered by compulsory health insurance either as a contributing member or as a dependent person (e.g., children). Opting out is not possible. Permanent residence is one of the most important factors for defining entitlement to health benefits, but Articles 15–18 of the Health Care and Health Insurance Act [7] set additional conditions under which a person is compulsorily insured [1, 2, 8].

According to the available data, 2,116,739 people were compulsorily insured in 2019, representing more than 99% of the population [1, 9]. About 0.14% (3345) people were uninsured at the end of 2020 [1, 9]. Most of them were temporarily

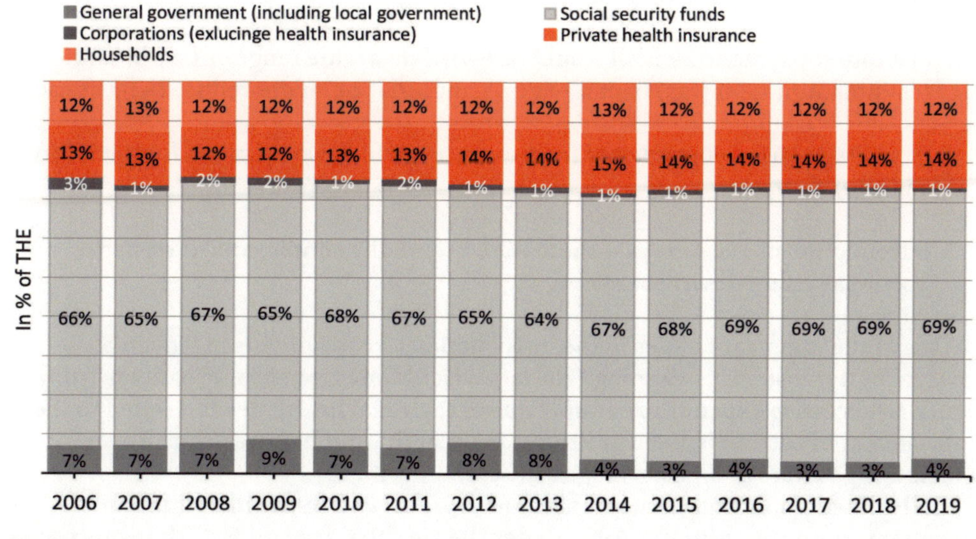

Figure 2.
Total health expenditure by functions and sources of funding, Slovenia, 2006-2019. Source: Zver HE, 2021 [5]; Statistical Office of the Republic of Slovenia, 2018 [8].

uninsured, for example, because they were waiting for their entitlement to pension or unemployment benefits to be recognised. The rest were mainly people who could not meet the formal residence requirements (e.g., undocumented migrants and ethnic minorities, such as the Roma population and homeless people). In addition, at the end of 2020, 15, 892 people had compulsory insurance but did not pay their contributions, which means that their entitlement to health services was suspended, and they could only access emergency services [1].

According to the Health Care and Health Insurance Act [7], there are 25 categories of insured persons. Each category has a different contribution rate, but contributions are mostly income-based. The first big group is employees (and their dependents), the second group includes the unemployed, other persons without a fixed income who are not registered as unemployed, pensioners, farmers, and the self-employed [1]. The National Institute for Employment pays the contributions for the unemployed; the state and/or municipalities for persons without income, prisoners, and war veterans. In addition, European regulations and bilateral agreements provide health insurance coverage for citizens from almost all EU countries. Special provisions apply to certain vulnerable groups [1, 7].

4. The introduction and development of complementary health insurance

Slovenia had historical experience with copayments since they existed already in the previous political and health system, which was in force until 1990. They were introduced in the early 1980s, mostly as flat rates on top of services. As the period of 1980s was marked by very high inflation rates, such an approach resulted in copayments becoming a negligible contribution (estimated only at around 1% of THE in 1989) as well as not an important burden on the patients. Still, this experience—together with the exceptions from copayments—fed directly into the solutions proposed by the new legislation adopted in 1992 [1, 10, 11].

When the legislation was being prepared in the period 1990–1992, different solutions to copayments were discussed. Considerations were given to the following options:

1. Flat rate copayments, which would be levied on a wide range of health services (counter argument was that any significant inflation might reduce their impact).

2. Percentage-based copayments (coinsurance), which would allow for flexibility and stratification.

3. Introduction of exceptions—these were eventually simply copied from the previous system described above.

One of the important issues in the introduction of copayments in Slovenia, however, is the absence of capping. The latter would prevent chronic patients from incurring excessive expenditure simply due to their real health needs, related to the management of their existing conditions. In turn, this might have been also one of the contributing factors to high coverage by the CHI [1, 10, 11].

CHI gained popularity, acceptance, and advocacy with the introduction of copayments into the system in 1992 under the Health Care and Health Insurance Act [7]. However, the most important regulations chronologically presented in the market development of CHI are listed below (**Table 1**) [1, 10, 11]. CHI served to

1992	The HCHI (1992), the Health Services Act (1992), and the Pharmacies Act (1992) enable the introduction of private financing (CHI as VHI is introduced in 1993).
1999	The Act amending the Health Care and Health Insurance Act (HCHI, 1998) established Vzajemna as a separate legal entity, completely separated from the HIIS.
2000	The Insurance Act (2000) declares that CHI serves the public interest; risk equalisation is introduced. In 2003, the White Paper (2003) is published and a reform proposal by the MoH calls for the abolition of CHI, which covers copayments.
2004	The Insurance Act (2004) again announced the introduction of a risk equalization mechanism. However, the mechanism was not implemented, and risk-based premiums were still allowed.
2005	The HCHI Amendment Act (2005) introduces community-based premiums for CHI to cover the copayments, risk equalisation CHI and penalties for late joiners to CHI (for every 12 months without CHI, calculated from the month a person becomes liable for paying the copayments, the premium increases by 3%, up to a maximum of 80%).
	Adriatic Slovenica (in October 2005) and Vzajemna (in December 2005) challenge the risk equalisation scheme in the Supreme Court. Adriatic Slovenica argues that the scheme would lead to higher average premiums and that this would undermine competition as it would lead to a monopoly in the long run; Vzajemna argues that the scheme does not consider the differences in the health status of persons insured with a given company and treats the companies unequally; the court upholds the government and confirms the legality of the adopted risk equalisation scheme.
2006	The HCHI Amendment Act (2005) comes into force; in response to the introduction of community rating, CHI premiums increase by 18%; a further 5% increase in premiums is attributed to rising health costs.
	In June 2006, Vzajemna complains to the EC about the following shortcomings of CHI covering user fees: (1) insurers offering CHI must be included in the compensation scheme; (2) the insurance supervisory authority must be informed of any change in the conditions of CHI; (3) any increase in these premiums must be confirmed in writing by a certified actuary and can only be made under the supervision of the appointed Authority; (4) the premiums for CHI to cover the access must be the same for all subscribers of a given insurer and the contracts must not be shorter than 1 year; (5) insurers may only terminate a CHI contract if the policyholder fails to pay the premiums; (6) the revenue generated by the CHI scheme may only be used for the implementation of this scheme; (7) half of all profits generated must be used for the implementation of the CHI scheme; (8) before an insurer enters the CHI market, it must obtain the written approval of the Minister of Health.
2007	In March 2007, the EC issued an official warning regarding Slovenia's health insurance legislation. The government had argued that CHI, which covers the copayments, despite its voluntary nature, was an integral part of the compulsory health insurance system and therefore a matter of public interest justifying government intervention to protect the general interest. The EC rejects this and argues that complementary health insurance is not a full or partial alternative to compulsory health insurance and cannot be considered part of the compulsory social security system based on EU law.
2011	The legislation on CHI is not changed and the EC refers Slovenia to the ECJ. The new reform proposal of the MoH. The modernisation of the health system by 2020 envisages the abolition of copayments and the introduction of a redefined, publicly financed benefits package.
2012	The Public Finance Balancing Act (2012) shifts costs from compulsory to complementary insurance (from public to private sector) which leads to a 13% increase in premiums for CHI.
	The ECJ confirms that Slovenian legislation on the CHI does not fully comply with the Directives on non-life insurance. The ruling concerns, among other things, the use of profits, systematic reporting, and prior authorisation; it does not concern risk equalisation.

Note: EC—the European Commission; ECJ—the European Court of Justice; CHI—complementary (voluntary) health insurance; HCHI—The Health Care and Health Insurance Amendment Act; MoH—Ministry of Health; VHI—voluntary health insurance.
Source: European Commission, 2012 [10]; Sagan A, Thomson S, 2016 [11].

Table 1.
Development and regulation of CHI in Slovenia, 1992–2012.

raise additional funds for health care in addition to the funds from the compulsory health insurance and served to diversify the sources of funding. Originally, there were two providers of CHI: HIIS, and Adriatic, a for-profit commercial provider [11, 12].

In 1993–1994, mainly large companies concluded collective agreements with CHI for their employees. After initial fears that a two-class medical system would emerge, this later became a matter of individual choice. However, it was argued that the introduction of the CHI system would put an end to unlimited entitlements and the use of the compulsory health insurance system, as consumers would have to raise additional funds [11, 12].

In 1998, the Health Care and Health Insurance Act [7] was amended in such a way that the HIIS had to separate its compulsory insurance and CHI. As a result, a new non-profit mutual insurance company, Vzajemna, was established, independent of the HIIS, which subsequently became the largest provider of CHI. Ever since CHI has been on the market, there have been clear signs of imbalances between the various CHI companies. The equity problems became apparent when CHI introduced a regressive element into the system due to its flat-rate premiums (i.e., not risk-based). At that time, premiums for CHI were not risk-based and two companies (Adriatic and Vzajemna) charged identical premiums [11, 12].

When the two commercial companies offering CHI entered the Slovenian market in 2004–2005, they launched an obvious advertising campaign for younger and healthier policyholders with risk-based premiums. CHI is regulated by the Insurance Supervisory Authority (premiums level) and the MoH (market entry, approval of initial premiums, risk equalisation procedure). It does not receive tax subsidies. The CHI market is subject to relatively strict regulation, and some argue that these rules violate EU regulations [11, 12].

In 2006, the amendment to the Health Care and Health Insurance Act 2005 [7] came into force. In response to the introduction of the Community Rating, premiums increased by 18% and by a further 5% due to rising health costs. In June 2006, Vzajemna complains to the European Commission (EC) about the shortcomings of CHI (**Table 1**). In 2007, the EC issued an official warning regarding Slovenia's health insurance legislation. The government had argued that CHI, which covers the copayments for most of the services in the basic benefit package, despite its voluntary nature, is an integral part of compulsory health insurance and a matter of public interest for the protection of the common good.

In 2011, EC took Slovenia to the European Court of Justice (ECJ) for failing to amend the CHI legislation. As a result, the MoH proposed to reform the health system by 2020 and abolish CHI with a redefined publicly funded benefits package. In 2012, the Public Finance Balancing Act was passed, resulting in a shift of costs from the public to the private sector and a 13% increase in CHI premiums to cover user fees [11]. The European Court of Justice confirms that Slovenian legislation on the CHI does not fully comply with the non-life insurance directives. The ruling concerns, among other things, the use of profits, systematic reporting, and prior authorisation; it does not concern risk equalisation [11]. After several reminders, EC decided to refer the issue of this non-life insurance (health insurance) to the ECJ, which resulted in a ruling by the ECJ declaring that the provision of CHI in Slovenia is in breach of the Non-Life Insurance Directive. No direct penalty was imposed, but the Slovenian government was ordered to put an end to the infringement and to inform EC of the decision [10].

5. Advantages and disadvantages of complementary health insurance

5.1 Complementary health insurance in economic crisis

Slovenia was hit by an economic crisis a little bit later than some EU countries, at the end of 2008, when the business orders from abroad began to decline and consequently, the unemployment started to increase. As 98% of all incomes for compulsory health insurance are represented by contributions paid from wages and other incomes by the population, these changes had a big impact on the health insurance income. To assure that compulsory health insurance can still cover all its expenditures, numerous measures had to be passed. Among these measures, CHI played an important role. Compared to 2010, in 2015 expenditure on compulsory health insurance increased by € 49.17 M or 2.3%, while expenditure on CHI increased by € 66.31 M or 16.3% (**Figure 3**).

The average annual growth rate of compulsory health insurance expenditure in this period was 0.46%, while CHI expenditure was 3.07%. The growth rate of CHI expenditure was, hence, seven times higher than the growth rate of compulsory health insurance.

Despite stricter business conditions and the same contribution rate and equal (or at least not lower) access of insured persons to health services, the HIIS must comply with the commitment of the Stability and Growth Pact adopted by the EU in 1998 and subsequently upgraded several times. The Stability and Growth Pact is a set of rules that ensure that countries in the European Union maintain sound public finances and coordinate fiscal policies. According to the rules, HIIS must ensure the balance of revenues and expenditures without borrowing. As this was simply not possible in times of economic crisis, HIIS adopted and implemented innovative measures in 2009 to ensure its stable business operation. In determining the measures, the focus was on finding reserves in the compulsory health insurance system, without compromising the access of insured persons to services and without changing the rights from compulsory health insurance. The measures were primarily aimed at lowering the prices

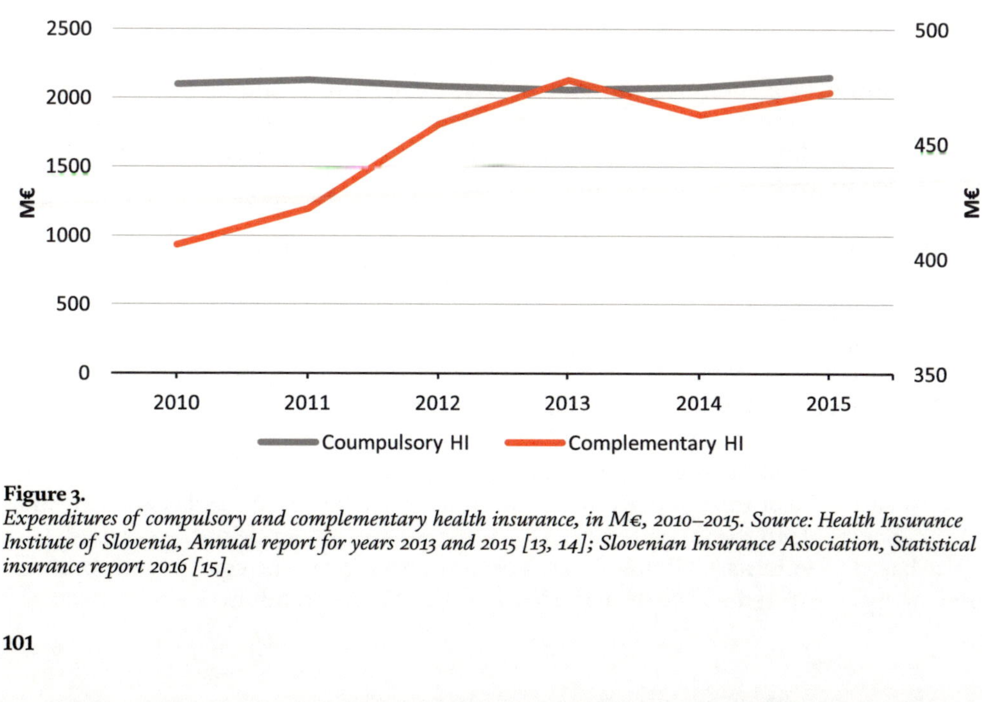

Figure 3.
Expenditures of compulsory and complementary health insurance, in M€, 2010–2015. Source: Health Insurance Institute of Slovenia, Annual report for years 2013 and 2015 [13, 14]; Slovenian Insurance Association, Statistical insurance report 2016 [15].

of health services and reducing the share of the price covered by compulsory health insurance and increasing the share of the price covered by CHI for medicines, medical devices, services, sickness benefits. The changes in the coverage shares happened at two levels.

The first transfer of financial obligations from compulsory onto CHI happened when HIIS passed the Decision on determining the percentage of the value of health services provided in compulsory health insurance, on 18 July 2009, namely for a spa treatment that does not represent the continuation of hospital treatment and for medicines from the interim list. The validity of the amendment to the resolution on determining the percentage of the value of health services provided in compulsory health insurance was extended to the whole of 2010. On 15 February 2010, HIIS additionally extended the reduction of the share of services at the expense of compulsory health insurance to the field of non-emergency ambulances, spa treatment other than hospital treatment, dental prosthetic services, and eye accessories for adults.

The second package of changes was brought about by the Fiscal Balance Act (2012) with the following measures:

Reduction of the share of the value of health services covered by compulsory health insurance (from 1 January 2013 onwards), meaning the transfer of the financial burden to CHI, namely:

- Around 90% of the value (instead of 95%) for organ transplants, the most demanding surgical procedures, regardless of the reason, treatment services abroad, intensive care, radiotherapy, dialysis, and other most demanding diagnostic, therapeutic and rehabilitation services,

- Around 80% of the value (instead of 85%) for health services related to the provision and treatment of reduced fertility and artificial insemination, sterilisation, and abortion; specialist outpatient, hospital, and spa services as a continuation of hospital treatment, except for injuries outside work, non-medical part of care in hospital and spa within the continuation of hospital treatment, except for injuries outside work, treatment of dental and oral diseases, medical devices, and injuries outside work,

- Around 70% of the value (instead of 75%) for specialist outpatient, hospital, and spa services as a continuation of hospital treatment and non-medical part of the hospital and spa care as a continuation of hospital treatment, medical devices related to the treatment of injuries outside work, medicines from the positive list.

The increase in complementary health insurance is evident also from the increase of the share of complementary health insurance expenditure in GDP between 2010 and 2015: while this share increased by 0.10 percentage points, the share of compulsory health insurance decreased by 0.22 percentage points.

5.2 Complementary health insurance and inequities

CHI is purchased by more than 95% of the population liable for co-insurance, which means 73% of the population. The premiums are flat-based and regressive and cover copayments in the range between 10% and 90% of the price of the services. Due to flat-based premiums, CHI has always been criticized from the equity viewpoint. In time, many adjustments have been made to the flat-based premium, such as coverage of costs of copayments for the socially vulnerable, who cannot afford to purchase CHI. Copayments are also covered for war veterans and prisoners. As the copayments are covered at the point of the service, the inequities caused by flat-based premiums are largely tackled, except for around 5% of the population right above the income limit, which would enable them to receive social benefits. For these citizens, the insurance is out of reach and might face higher unmet needs.

Since 2006, the share of CHI in total household consumption levelled around 2.9%. In 2012, the regressive nature of CHI premiums was importantly limited, when automatic coverage of CHI claims for all socially vulnerable populations from the central budget was introduced (**Figure 4**).

Due to the widely defined basic benefits package, covered by two financial sources, the demand for additional services, that are not included in the basic benefit package, is very low. The out-of-pocket payments are, consequently, the lowest in the European region and amounted to 12% according to the last available data from 2018.

5.3 Complementary health insurance and risk selection

In Slovenia, a system of risk equalisation and the creation of an efficient model for the long-term sustainability of the health care financing system was prepared by the MoH and included in the law in 2005 [7, 12, 17]. Risk equalisation or compensation schemes are necessary to support community-rated health insurance and were created for the market CHI. Basically, health insurers receive credits or subsidies from a national fund or authority to compensate for the additional costs of insuring older and less healthy members. The Health Care and Health Insurance Act in Article 23 regulates the basket of health benefits for a compulsorily insured person [7], albeit very substantial, from 100% to 10% of the value of the healthcare service for most adult insured persons; payment of the difference or balance up to 100% of the value of the healthcare service is the responsibility of the insured person who received the healthcare service (also depending on the type of treatment or activity) [17]. To prevent 'cream-skimming', companies have been obliged to participate in risk

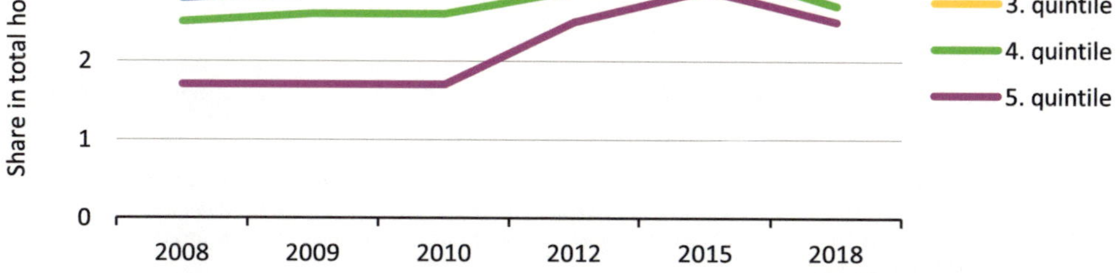

Figure 4.
CHI expenditure as share of total household consumption, according to income quintiles, 2008–2018. Source: Zver et al. [16].

equalisation to compensate for differences in health care costs between insurance companies [7, 12].

Quite restrictive legislation [7] stipulates that insurers are obliged to cover the costs of all publicly financed health services. Children are exempt from the copayments and therefore do not need CHI. CHI appears to be compulsory for adults, as they must pay penalties if they do not take out CHI once they become liable for the copayments. For each full year (12 months) that they do not have CHI, the penalty is 3% of the premium. The maximum penalty is 80% of the premium [17, 18]. The uniform flat premium for all CHI-insured persons established by the Health Care and Health Insurance Act [7] is independent of gender, age, or health status. However, equality is guaranteed between the different providers of CHI and between the insured person and the insurance conditions of CHI regarding the duration and termination of CHI contracts (**Table 2**) [12].

The monthly basic insurance premium for the three companies in the Slovenian market of CHI shows a sustained upward trend over the period 2006–2019, despite a slight price decrease from 2013 to 2014 (**Figure 5**). Between 2006 and 2013, the premium increased by €93 per insurance policy [12, 20]. Apparently, Generali and Triglav zdravje are slightly higher than Vzajemna, which could be a form of risk selection [19, 20].

The experience with risk equalisation shows that all three companies make regular payments to CHI, as would be appropriate given their risk profiles. However, these payments are quite small, amounting to only €12 M in 2014. This corresponds to about 3% of the total premium income [19, 20].

The simplest risk adjustment factors used to balance premium risk are based on age and gender. They are easy to collect and monitor, but they are a poor measure of expected health care costs [21]. Improving the risk equalisation formula should be a focus of government action to ensure that the market CHI functions efficiently [20].

5.4 Complementary health insurance and administration costs

In general, although monthly basic insurance premiums fell slightly from 2013 to 2016, they have shown a sustained upward trend in recent years. It seems that the austerity measures during the economic crisis had little impact on the price level (**Figure 5**). To understand the reason for the escalation of premium costs, it is useful to examine the relationship between premium income and claims costs. This helps in analysing the efficiency of CHI in financing health care. The discrepancy between revenue and claims costs shows the transaction costs of using CHI for this key role in health care financing. If this discrepancy increases, it indicates inefficiency as the same number of people is insured but with higher administrative costs. Moreover,

	Triglav zdravje	Vzajemna	Generali (Adriatic)
Basic premium	€ 35.55	€ 34.60*	€ 34.50

*Note: *Due to the circumstances of COVID-19, the premium CHI in December 2021 was €12.1 instead of €34.6, as Vzajemna returned €22.5 to policyholders. The average monthly CHI premium was thus €32.72 in 2021, but rose again to €34.6 in January 2022, as the other two CHI companies returned profits to shareholders in the form of dividends. Source: e-Zavarovanja, 2022 [19].*

Table 2.
Monthly premiums for CHI (€), April 2022.

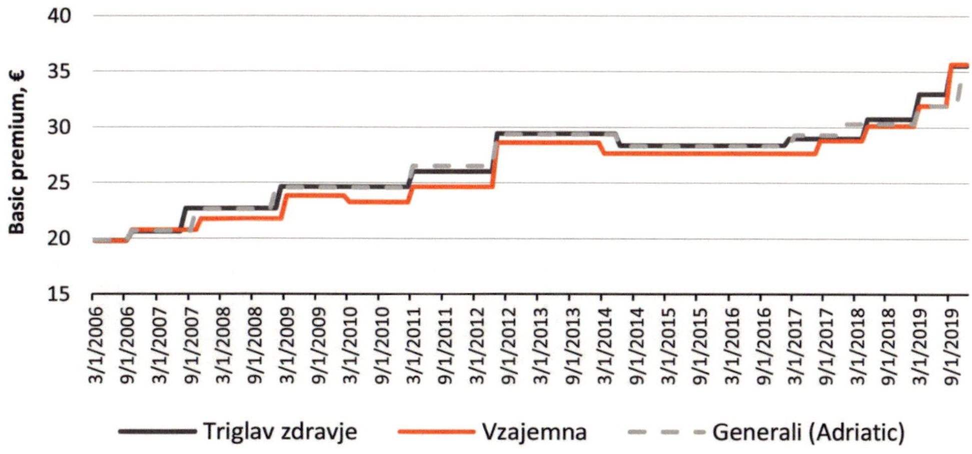

Figure 5.
Monthly premiums for CHI (€), March 2016—December 2019. Source: Data from CHI companies (authors' own calculations).

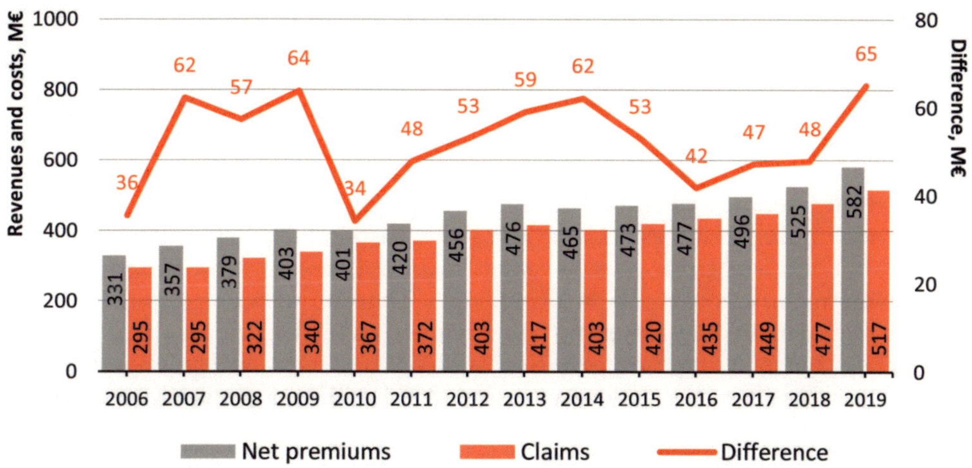

Figure 6.
Revenues and costs in the markets of CHI €, 2006-2019. Source: Slovenian Insurance Supervisory Authority, Annual Report for the years 2007–2020 [22–35] (authors' own calculations).

in due course, this may undermine the affordability of CHI, especially for poorer households [20].

Figure 6 shows how claims costs increased between 2007 and 2013 and then decreased slightly in 2014 (due to lower reserve costs, partly due to government pricing policies and covered benefits). Premium income has generally increased since 2006 (with slight decreases in 2010 and 2014). The difference between premiums and claims rose sharply before the crisis, reaching a peak of €64 M in 2009. As a result of the crisis, the premiums declined slightly in 2010, while claims kept on increasing, resulting in the lowest difference between both (€34 M in 2010). In the next 4 years, the revenues from premiums kept on increasing and the difference almost reached the pre-crisis level again in 2014. Another drop in the difference between revenues and claims can be observed in 2016 and 2019, the difference was again back to €65 M. [20, 22–35].

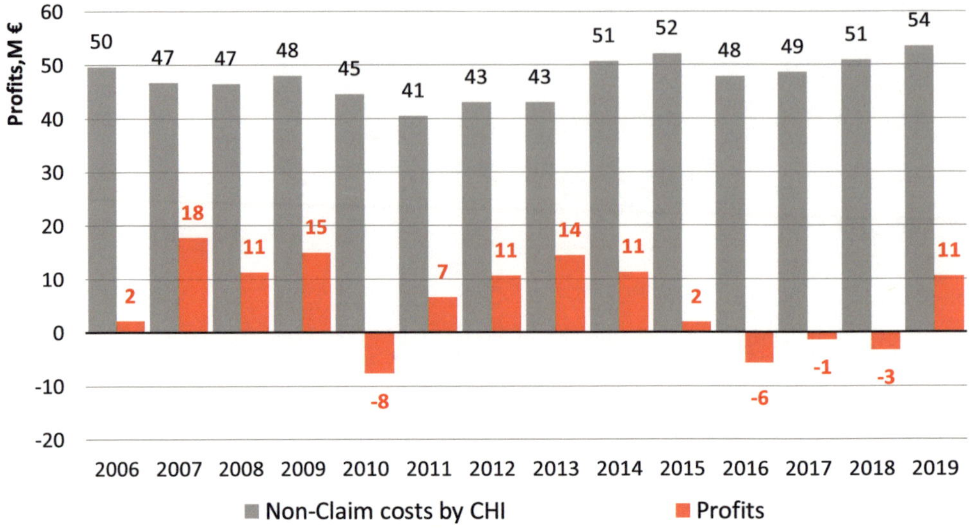

Figure 7.
Profits and non-claims costs in the markets of CHI, 2006–2019. Source: Slovenian Insurance Supervisory Authority, Annual Report for the years 2007–2020 [22–35].

Figure 7 shows a breakdown of the difference between premium income and non-claims expenditure, suggesting that much of this is due to actual operating costs rather than profits. However, the official profit figures may not fully reflect the difference between revenues and costs [20, 22–35]. However, compared to other countries that provide similar resources to CHI, transaction costs in Slovenia are very low [20]. This may not be too surprising, as Slovenian insurers do not purchase services and should therefore have lower administrative costs. There are also concerns that new solvency requirements could push up transaction costs further, although the extent is not yet fully known. Rising transaction costs should be a focus of regulation to ensure that CHI remains affordable for everyone and that the CHI market is administratively efficient [20, 22–35].

It should also focus on better monitoring so that the market is more transparent for regulatory authorities and consumers. In a truly competitive market, insurers would automatically correct prices downwards when their cost base is reduced. A helpful piece of regulation would be to set a minimum claims ratio so that insurers must spend a minimum share of premium income on health care costs. This would limit transaction costs and help secure affordability in the CHI market. The government should also tighten reporting requirements [20].

Although the administrative costs of CHI are low by international standards, CHI on the other hand incurs transaction costs related to insurers' profits and administrative costs, and indirectly to the costs of government regulation. The main risk of CHI is that transaction costs will continue to increase over time, reducing the administrative efficiency and affordability of this option, especially due to the new solvency requirements [20].

5.5 Complementary health insurance and efficiency

An increase in the efficiency of the health care system in Slovenia had been one of the declarative goals of the introduction of the CHI. It was supposed to reduce the 'unnecessary' demand for health services while also raising some additional financial resources for its functioning. One of the reasons for such reasoning lies in the fact that the structure of expenditures of CHI by categories is significantly different from compulsory health insurance. Namely, around 45% of the CHI expenditures are for the reimbursement of copayments on medicines (cf. the expenditures on medicines represent only 11.7% of the expenses of HIIS [36].

One of the disadvantages of CHI, which is rarely mentioned and discussed, is the impact of CHI on the efficiency of health services provision. As discussed above, the levels of copayments differ for different services. While they amount to 10% of the price for most important services, they can amount to as much as 90% of the price for services, less important for health (such as non-urgent transportation). While HIIS as a single provider of compulsory health insurance restricts the health care providers and pays the volume of their services up to a defined plan, the private health insurers offering CHI have no such restrictions. Intuitively, the providers can hence provide an unlimited number of less important services as they are 90% covered by CHI, resulting in less efficient and less cost-effective care provision. While a study, confirming such a theory, has not been conducted yet, the logic of the idea remains.

Another disadvantage of CHI to which not enough attention has been paid is surely its stabilisation role. As discussed in other sections of this chapter, CHI had a huge stabilisation impact in an economic crisis, buffering the negative impacts of higher unemployment. Resulting in a higher premium, the CHI managed to alleviate the impact of the lower incomes and contributions to compulsory health insurance. On the other hand, this enabled the health system, HIIS, and health care providers not to implement organisational changes, cost-effective measures, or increases in efficiency. The waste in the system remained the same, the outcomes are still not discussed and measured, and necessary reforms that would put the patient in the centre of integrated care still seem non-urgent in spite of long waiting times.

As had been established with a specially commissioned analysis of the performance of the Slovenian health system in 2015 by the World Health Organization (WHO) and the European Observatory on Health Systems and Policies [37], CHI played an important role in buffering the shocks experienced by the health system in the times of austerity (the period between 2009–2010 and 2014). These shocks were reflected primarily in a rapid decline in paid contributions against compulsory health insurance as unemployment rose dramatically between the end of 2009 and the first half of 2012[1] [38]. In that period, the Government intervened at various levels to stabilize public finance (e.g., by reducing salaries in the public sector) but in doing so it also further reduced the contributions to health insurance. HIIS acted in two ways—partly their payments were positively affected by the reduction in salaries, but they still reduced payments to hospitals by 15% in 2 years and they shifted some expenditure to CHI. This was possible as HIIS had the authority of establishing the percentage coverage of a range of services, which attracted copayments. Such an approach reduced pressure on HIIS and introduced further 'cost-sharing' between HIIS and the insurance providers of CHI.

[1] In September 2008, the number of unemployed was at its lowest level since January 1992 at 59,303, only to rise in the wake of the crisis to a peak of 129,843 unemployed in January 2014, an increase of 219% [38].

6. Health policy and complementary health insurance

CHI has remained one of the main focuses of health policy in Slovenia since its introduction. As much as it has been praised at its introduction and as much as it has been criticized all along the way, no government so far was able to significantly modify it in either way (e.g., either abolishing it or turning it into a more extensive mixed mutual health insurance). The first serious and organized attempt had been done with the Health Reform proposal published in 2003 [39].

According to that initiative and reform, the CHI would be entirely integrated into the compulsory health insurance and would thus cease to exist. After a fierce debate and controversies within the government itself, it was not implemented. There were two more attempts, which were systematically carried out by the Government, more precisely by the MoH. The first of the two was the initiative of the MoH in 2012 to seek reconstruction of this insurance and explore the possibility of it extending its scope. A policy dialogue was organised together with the European Observatory on Health Systems and Policies (Observatory). It resulted in the conclusions of not liberalising the market of these insurance and not extending their role to additional services, for example, long-term care. Finally, in the MoH term between 2014 and 2018, the minister was focused strongly on transforming the CHI into parallel compulsory insurance, which would be stratified in contributions by the income brackets, established by the IRS. This initiative ran close to its completion, but there were significant reserves. One of the important ones was in the report commissioned by the MoH to the Observatory and WHO, where the main conclusion was that the CHI contributed to the stabilisation of health financing in the times of austerity and shortages in public funding (see also above and [40]).

Remaining at very high levels of coverage and effectively covering around 83% of the total population and around 95% of those who are obliged to pay copayments it represents an important instrument for raising additional financial resources and collecting them in a transgenerational manner. The latter is the main factor why the CHI remains an asset and not a burden for the decision- and policymakers.

7. Conclusion

Although CHI had not been envisaged as such at the very beginning of the transitional reforms in Slovenia from the old political, social, and economic system to a new one in 1990–1992, it has taken ground over the past 30 years. This development occurred despite several attempts at abolishing it or transforming it into a different conceptual framework (especially in view of the need for a system approach to long-term care insurance). It has proven to be robust, and it has served to the purpose of buffering some potential negative fallout of the economic crisis from 2009 to 2014. Furthermore, contrary to the most significant and often repeated criticism, namely, that it was a regressive type of health insurance, it has proven to have a good level of transgenerational solidarity. Flat-rate premiums were the trigger to claims of regressivity, but the fact that a healthy population of persons in their 20s and 30s paying the same premiums as those above 65 years of age clearly shows an important lever for solidarity. A very high level of coverage through the inclusion of much of the adult population in the CHI enables such a situation. The intervention with which the Government around 15 years ago protected persons, who for economic reasons cannot pay for the premiums of the CHI serves as another example of solidarity and social correction of socio-economic differences. The more covert aspects of inefficiency, namely, the structure of the provided services and delay in cost-effectiveness measures, are visible only upon a systematic understanding of the health care financing system and therefore rarely discussed and put forward. Generally, productivity is dealt with only indirectly through the pricing of reimbursement criteria set up by HIIS, which has not been updated and endorsed by the medical professional societies.

The most adverse effect of a potential abolishment of CHI would very likely be a system of uninsurable copayments, which would affect the vulnerable layers of the population in Slovenia to a much more significant degree than the flat-rate premiums, with all the introduced adjustments for socially vulnerable, do. We can conclude that amidst strong pressures for either its abolishment or its expansion, the CHI in Slovenia has proven to be an important resource for the stabilisation of health expenditure. Despite it being a private insurance as it is paid after taxes, it bears a very strong public and social component.

List of abbreviations

WHO	World Health Organization
CHI	Complementary Health Insurance
MoH	Ministry of Health
VHI	Voluntary Health Insurance
THE	Total Health Expenditures
GDP	Gross Domestic Product
HIIS	Health Insurance Institute of Slovenia
ECJ	European Court of Justice
EC	European Commission

Author details

Tit Albreht[1,2,3], Marjeta Kuhar[1,4] and Valentina Prevolnik Rupel[5,6*]

1 National Institute of Public Health, Ljubljana, Slovenia

2 Faculty of Medicine, University of Maribor, Maribor, Slovenia

3 Faculty of Medicine, University of Ljubljana, Ljubljana Slovenia

4 University of Ljubljana, Ljubljana, Slovenia

5 Faculty of Social Science, Institute for Economic Research, Ljubljana, Slovenia

6 DOBA Faculty, Maribor, Slovenia

*Address all correspondence to: katka.rupel@gmail.com

References

[1] Zgrablić B. The equalization scheme of the residual voluntary health insurance in Slovenia. Ars Mathematica Contemporanea. 2015;**8**(1):225-234. DOI: 10.26493/1855-3974.667.fec

[2] Albreht T, Turk E, Toth M, Ceglar J, Marn S, Pribaković Brinovec R, et al. Slovenia: Health system review. Health Systems in Transition. 2009;**11**(3):1-168. Available from: http://www.euro.who.int/en/home/projects/observatory/publications/health-system-profiles-hits/full-list-of-hits [Accessed: April 17, 2022]

[3] Fiscal Balance Act. Official Gazette of the Republic of Slovenia, No 40/2012 with amendments, 11 May 2012 [Internet]. 2012. Available from: http://www.pisrs.si/Pis.web/pregledPredpisa?id=ZAKO6388 [Accessed: April 06, 2022]

[4] Slovenian Insurance Association. Statistical insurance report for year 2015 [Internet]. 2016. Available from: https://www.zav-zdruzenje.si/wp-content/uploads/2017/10/Statisti%C4%8Dni-zavarovalni%C5%A1ki-bilten-2015.pdf [Accessed: April 03, 2022]

[5] Zver E, Nagode M, Srakar A. Access to health care and long-term care. In: Gabrijelčič Blenkuš M et al. editors. Inequalities in Health: Future Challenges for Intersectoral Cooperation [Internet]. National Institute of Public Health Slovenia; 2021. Available from: https://www.nijz.si/en/publikacije/inequalities-in-health-future-challenges-intersectoral-cooperation [Accessed: April 03, 2022]

[6] Prevolnik Rupel V. ESPN Thematic Report on Inequalities in Access to Healthcare Slovenia, 2018. Brussels: European Commission [Internet]; 2018. Available from: https://www.google.com/url?sa=t&rct=j&q=&esrc=s&source=web&cd=&ved=2ahUKEwi_zdW2pc7xAhWGOuwKHY4DfYQFjABegQIBBAD&url=https%3A%2F%2Fec.europa.eu%2Fsocial%2FBlobServlet%3FdocId%3D20347%26langId%3Den&usg=AOvVaw2lLlcbjtFq1B3Qy_rs68uE [Accessed: April 06, 2022]

[7] Albreht T, Polin K, Pribaković Brinovec R, Kuhar M, Poldrugovac M, Ogrin Rehberger P, et al. Slovenia: Health system review. Health Systems in Transition. 2021;**23**(1):i-188

[8] Institute for Macroeconomic Analysis and Development. Economic issues 2019 [Internet]. 2020. Available from: https://www.umar.gov.si/fileadmin/user_upload/publikacije/izzivi/2019/angleski/a_EI_2019_cel.pdf [Accessed: April 10, 2022]

[9] Sagan A, Thomson S. Voluntary health insurance in Europe: Country experience. Obs Stud Ser [Internet]. 2016;**42**:157-161. Available from: http://www.euro.who.int/__data/assets/pdf_file/0011/310799/Voluntary-health-insurance-Europe-country-experience.pdf?ua=1 [Accessed: April 10, 2022]

[10] Statistical Office of the Republic of Slovenia. Health expenditure and sources of funding, Slovenia, 2018 [Intranet]. 2019. Available from: https://www.stat.si/StatWeb/en/News/Index/8916 [Accessed: September 01, 2021]

[11] Health Insurance Institute of Slovenia. Annual report for year 2019 [Internet]. 2020. Available from: https://www.zzzs.si/zzzs-api/e-gradiva/vsa-gradiva/?vrsta=BR39ZT328 [Accessed: April 06, 2022]

[12] Martin P, Del Sol M. The uncertain and differentiated impact

of EU law on national (Private) Health Insurance Regulations. Priv Heal Insur Eur Union. 2021:85-127. DOI: 10.1007/978-3-030-54355-6_4

[13] Health Care and Health Insurance Act. Official Gazette of the Republic of Slovenia, No 72/2006 with amendments, 12 February 1992. [Internet]. 1992. Available from: http://pisrs.si/Pis.web/pregledPredpisa?id=ZAKO213 [Accessed: April 04, 2022]

[14] European Commission. Judgment of the Court (Eighth Chamber) of 26 January 2012 - European Commission v Republic of Slovenia (Case C-185/11) [Internet]. 2012. Available from: https://eur-lex.europa.eu/legal-content/en/TXT/?uri=CELEX:62011CJ0185 [Accessed: April 17, 2022]

[15] Health Insurance Institute of Slovenia. Annual report for year 2015 [Internet]. 2016. Available from: https://www.zzzs.si/zzzs-api/e-gradiva/vsa-gradiva/?vrsta=BR39ZT328 [Accessed: April 06, 2022]

[16] Zver EH. Ekonomika zdravstva, Viri in izdatki za zdravstvo v Sloveniji in državah EU (English: Health economics, resources, and expenditure on health care in Slovenia and EU countries) [Internet]. Institute for Macroeconomic Analysis and Development. 2021. Available from: https://www.nijz.si/sites/www.nijz.si/files/uploaded/ekonomika_zdravstva_viri_in_izdatki_za_zdravstvo_v_sloveniji_in_eu_eva_zver_24.5.pdf [Accessed: May 24, 2021]

[17] e-Zavarovanja. Complementary health insurance [Internet]. 2022. Available from: https://www.dopolnilnozavarovanje.si/pogosta-vprasanja/kaj-je-dopolnilno-zdravstveno-zavarovanje/ [Accessed: April 17, 2022]

[18] Ellis RP. Risk Adjustment in Health Care Markets: Concepts and Applications. Financing Health Care: New Ideas for a Changing Society. Weinheim: Wiley-VCH Verlag; 2008. pp. 177- 222. DOI: 10.1002/9783527611294.ch8

[19] Slovenian Insurance Supervision Agency. Annual report for year 2007 [Internet]. 2008. Available from: https://www.a-zn.si/wp-content/uploads/letno_porocilo-2007.pdf [Accessed: April 10, 2022]

[20] Thomas S, Thomson S, Evetovits T. Making sense of complementary health insurance, Final report WHO [Intranet]. 2015. Available from: https://www.euro.who.int/__data/assets/pdf_file/0011/336395/Making-Sense-of-Complementary-Health-Insurance-report-Slovenia.pdf [Accessed: April 17, 2022]

[21] Slovenian Insurance Supervision Agency. Annual report for year 2008 [Internet]. 2009. Available from: https://www.a-zn.si/wp-content/uploads/letno_porocilo-2008.pdf [Accessed: April 10, 2022]

[22] Slovenian Insurance Supervision Agency. Annual report for year 2009 [Internet]. 2010. Available from: https://www.a-zn.si/wp-content/uploads/letno_porocilo-2009.pdf [Accessed: April 10, 2022]

[23] Slovenian Insurance Supervision Agency. Annual report for year 2010 [Internet]. 2011. Available from: https://www.a-zn.si/wp-content/uploads/letno_porocilo-2010.pdf [Accessed: April 10, 2022]

[24] Slovenian Insurance Supervision Agency. Annual report for year 2011 [Internet]. 2012. Available from: https://www.a-zn.si/wp-content/uploads/letno_porocilo-2011.pdf [Accessed: April 10, 2022]

[25] Slovenian Insurance Supervision Agency. Annual report for year 2012 [Internet]. 2013. Available from: https://www.a-zn.si/wp-content/uploads/letno_porocilo-2012.pdf [Accessed: April 10, 2022]

[26] Slovenian Insurance Supervision Agency. Annual report for year 2013 [Internet]. 2014. Available from: https://www.a-zn.si/wp-content/uploads/letno_porocilo-2013.pdf [Accessed: April 10, 2022]

[27] Slovenian Insurance Supervision Agency. Annual report for year 2014 [Internet]. 2015. Available from: https://www.a-zn.si/wp-content/uploads/letno_porocilo-2014.pdf [Accessed: April 10, 2022]

[28] Slovenian Insurance Supervision Agency. Annual report for year 2015 [Internet]. 2016. Available from: https://www.a-zn.si/wp-content/uploads/letno_porocilo-2015.pdf [Accessed: April 10, 2022]

[29] Slovenian Insurance Supervision Agency. Annual report for year 2016 [Internet]. 2017. Available from: https://www.a-zn.si/wp-content/uploads/letno_porocilo-2016.pdf [Accessed: April 10, 2022]

[30] Slovenian Insurance Supervision Agency. Annual report for year 2017 [Internet]. 2018. Available from: https://www.a-zn.si/wp-content/uploads/letno_porocilo-2017.pdf [Accessed: April 10, 2022]

[31] Slovenian Insurance Supervision Agency. Annual report for year 2018 [Internet]. 2019. Available from: https://www.a-zn.si/wp-content/uploads/AZN-Letno-porocilo-2018.pdf [Accessed: April 10, 2022]

[32] Slovenian Insurance Supervision Agency. Annual report for year 2019 [Internet]. 2020. Available form: https://www.a-zn.si/wp-content/uploads/AZN-Letno-porocilo-2019.pdf [Accessed: April 10, 2022]

[33] Slovenian Insurance Supervision Agency. Annual report for year 2020 [Internet]. 2021. Available from: https://www.a-zn.si/wp-content/uploads/letno_porocilo-2020.pdf [Accessed: April 10, 2022]

[34] Health Insurance Institute of Slovenia. Annual report for year 2021 [Internet]. 2022. Available from: https://www.zzzs.si/?id=126&detail=12ED7829B4BE74DCC12587F80044EABD [Accessed: April 10, 2022]

[35] Thomson S, Evetovits T. Preučitev smiselnosti dopolnilnega zdravstvenega zavarovanja (English: A study on the rationale for the complementary health insurance). WHO Europe and European Observatory on Health Systems and policies, October 2015 [Internet]. 2015. Available from: chrome-extension://efaidnbmnnnibpcajpcglclefindmkaj/viewer.html?pdfurl=https%3A%2F%2Fwww.gov.si%2Fassets%2Fministrstva%2FMZ%2FDOKUMENTI%2FOrganizacija-zdravstvenega-varstva%2FAnaliza-zdravstvenega-sistema-v-Sloveniji%2FSLO_Preucitev-upravicenosti-dopolnilnega-zdravstvenega-zavarovanja.pdf&clen=963295 [Accessed: April 22, 2022]

[36] Employment Service of the Republic of Slovenia. Statistical data on unemployment in Slovenia, monthly statistics from 1992 to 2022 [Internet] 2022. Available from: https://www.ess.gov.si/_files/14934/Mesecno_gibanje_BO_1992-2022.xls [Accessed: April 24, 2022]

[37] Keber D, Leskovar B, Petrič V-K. Zdravstvena reforma: pravičnost, dostopnost, kakovost, učinkovitost:

osnutek (English: Health Reform: fairness, access, quality, and performance: a draft). Ljubljana, Slovenija: Vlada Republike Slovenije, Ministrstvo za zdravje; 2003

[38] Klemenčič Š. Financiranje sistema zdravstvenega varstva na temelju solidarnosti in socialne pravičnosti (English: Funding of the health care system based on solidarity and social justice). Master's thesis. Kranj: University of Maribor, Faculty of Organisational Sciences [Intranet]. 2018. Available from: https://dk.um.si/Dokument.php?id=130631&lang=eng [Accessed: April 06, 2022]

[39] Health Insurance Institute of Slovenia. Annual report for year 2020 [Internet]. 2021. Available from: https://www.zzzs.si/zzzs-api/e-gradiva/podrobnosti/?detail=A998991F0F548B4BC125868C0040BA61&id=126&cHash=e92a64e133c52989eb1e41a24796ecc6 [Accessed: April 06, 2022]

[40] Health Insurance Institute of Slovenia. Annual report for year 2013 [Internet]. 2014. Available from: https://www.zzzs.si/zzzs-api/e-gradiva/vsa-gradiva/?vrsta=BR39ZT328 [Accessed: April 06, 2022]

Chapter 7

Voluntary Private Health Insurance Demand by Older People in a National Health Service, the Case of Portugal

Aida Isabel Tavares

Abstract

The Portuguese health system is mainly described as a National Health Service (NHS). In parallel with the NHS, there are some Bismarkean features, like those arising from the existence of occupation-based health insurance. On top of these two layers of health insurance coverage, there is a market for private health insurance on a voluntary basis, which older people may not be able to access. The purpose of this work is to estimate the main determinants for older people in Portugal to buy private health insurance since no previous studies have been published. We use data collected by the National Health Survey of 2014 and estimate a multivariate probit. The main results are aligned with previous studies relating to income, education, and age. The role of the health status and behavior explaining the demand for private health insurance, in our results are mixed. People benefiting from parallel occupation-based insurance schemes are less likely to have a private voluntary health insurance policy. The results obtained in this work confirm that there is some inequality in health care access, to the detriment of older people.

Keywords: voluntary health insurance, determinants, older people, NHS, Portugal

1. Introduction

The Portuguese health system is mainly described as a National Health Service (NHS), following the Beveridge tradition, with universal coverage and mandatory participation. In parallel with the NHS, there are some Bismarkean features, such as those arising from the existence of occupation-based health insurance, which are also mandatory or quasi-mandatory. On top of these two layers of health insurance coverage, there is a market for private health insurance on a voluntary basis. This insurance is both supplementary and complementary to the NHS. People may be interested in buying a health insurance policy because it gives them faster access to health care, lets them choose the provider and enjoy a better experience when admitted to a hospital, and have access to services not included in the NHS, such as dental care [1].

Over the last 6 years, health care expenditure on private VHI in Portugal as a percentage of GDP has been less than 0.5% and it has been about 5% of current health expenditure [2]. Despite this trend, voluntary private health insurance in Portugal grew by about 3.5% between 2012 and 2015 [3].

The insurance market is characterized by asymmetric information [4, 5] expressed by moral hazard [6] and by adverse selection [7]. A moral hazard happens after the insurance contract has been signed and it refers to the situation where the insured person uses more health care services than they would need. On the other hand, adverse selection happens before the insurance contract has been signed, when the insurance company cannot assess the risk type of individual purchasing the insurance. This individual may be a low health risk, so they will be mainly healthy and generate low health care spending, or they may be high risk and will generate high health care spending. If the adverse selection does not take place, then low-risk individuals might prefer to buy the insurance and this is called advantageous or propitious selection [8], which is beneficial to insurance companies. This situation is often explained by a person's risk preferences. Healthy people tend to be risk-averse and so they choose to buy VHI [9, 10].

Older people are often considered as high health risk individuals, who are very likely to have more health problems than younger individuals, have higher medical expenditures, and raise the claims paid by insurance companies [11]. Not only do these people have more health problems, but insurance companies face moral hazards and adverse selection issues that result in the overuse of health care and the payment of excessive claims. For these reasons, older people are not usually the customers desired by insurance companies.

The Portuguese health insurance market is not as highly regulated as it is in other countries, because health insurance is voluntary and the NHS has universal coverage. So, insurance companies can adopt several strategies to prevent or mitigate moral hazard and adverse selection [12] and to reduce paying out excessive claims. One strategy could involve the eligibility requirements excluding people older than 65. Even though this cream-skimming strategy discriminates against older people, there is a small health insurance market for older people in Portugal. In the last available National Health Survey, conducted in 2014, of the 5,701 people older than 65 interviewed, 5.8% of them stated they had a voluntary health insurance policy.

The purpose of this work is to estimate the main determinants for older people in Portugal to take out private health insurance since no previous studies have been published and there may be differences across European countries [13, 14]. We use data collected by the 2014 National Health Survey and we estimate a multivariate probit. We also compute the marginal effects associated with the most important variables. This analysis provides insights for designing health and social policies that will reduce the inequality in health care access that may be generated by differences in health insurance coverage.

1.1 Demand determinants for voluntary private health insurance

The factors explaining the demand for VHI are well discussed in the literature. While Outreville [15] focused on the demand for insurance in general, [16, 17] have looked at the demand for VHI and reviewed the determinants for buying it; [1] outlined these determinants for the EU countries. The explanatory factors include the demographic and economic determinants (also referred to as socioeconomic status), that is, gender, age, education, income, marital status, employment status, and other characteristics [11, 13, 16–19]. In general, we can say that the likelihood of purchasing VPHI increases with age, income, education, being employed, and living in urban areas. The results are not conclusive for determinants, such as gender, family composition, and being a pensioner.

In Europe, where health systems tend to be mandatory and offer universal coverage, the determinants for holding a private VHI differ between countries [13, 14]. Regarding Portugal, an empirical study performed almost 20 years ago [20], concluded that the VHI buyers were most likely young, self-employed, living in urban areas, and receiving a middle to high income, thus leaving out older people.

The focus on the demand for private VHI by older people has been much less studied because it is known that as we age, the likelihood of having this type of insurance decreases [21]. Four empirical works should be mentioned that are concerned exclusively with older people and use the data collected by SHARE – Survey of Health, Aging, and Retirement in Europe [18, 13, 14, 19]. In general, being female, having had a good education, and receiving a higher income increases the demand for private VHI by older people.

Special attention is often given to the role of the health status and health behavior since there are proxies for the individual healthrisk type [22]. Health status can be measured by self-assessed health and the presence (or the number) of chronic diseases [18, 23], while health behavior can be proxied by body mass index or being overweight [24], and by smoking decisions [25].

The theory predicts that high-risk individuals are more likely to have health insurance, that is, adverse selection exists in health insurance. However, there are no conclusive empirical results regarding the relationship between individual risk variables and having a VHI policy [16]. This means that advantageous selection is a possibility, where low-risk type people choose to buy health insurance [23, 26].

The empirical results regarding indicators of health status and health-related behavior are mixed. Some studies have found that people reporting better health are more likely to have voluntary health insurance, supporting the hypothesis of advantageous selection [11, 12, 14, 18, 23, 27–29]; other authors found no significant correlation [27, 30]; and still, others found that healthy people tend to have VHI less often, as predicted by adverse selection hypothesis [11, 12, 14, 19].

In most studies, indicators of chronic diseases are found to be insignificant when explaining the demand for VHI [29, 31, 32]. Few works have reported a positive correlation between suffering from chronic diseases and having private health insurance [18, 23].

The relationship between health-related behaviors and private VHI coverage has been studied less and the results are mixed [14]. While some studies find that smokers are less likely to have VHI [27, 33], others find the opposite [18]. The results are similarly mixed for overweight people. It may be found that being overweight is associated with lower odds of taking out VHI or more likely [24].

1.2 Overview of the Portuguese health system

The Portuguese Health System, created in 1979, is defined as a National Health Service; it is mainly financed through taxes and is a universal coverage system. This means it covers all residents and most medical services.

In parallel with the NHS, there are occupation-based health insurance schemes. These include the public insurance schemes that cover civil servants (called ADSE), the armed forces (called ADM), and also private insurance that covers bank employees (called SAMS), among others. There are other, smaller, occupation-based health insurance plans. All the social contributions under these professional insurance policies are income based.

The Portuguese health system comprises conventional private health insurance and it is non-compulsory. Voluntary health insurance (VHI) provides faster access to appointments and treatments, which are also provided by the NHS, or provides access to services not covered by the NHS, such as dental care.

According to NHS rules, people should be registered with an NHS general practitioner, for primary care, and access to specialists in the NHS is controlled by general practitioner gatekeeping. However, people covered by insurance have direct access to specialists (provided by the private sector) according to the rules of the insurance, and private physicians can refer patients to NHS hospitals. So, having an insurance policy on top of NHS coverage has some advantages when it comes to accessing health care services [3]. These reasons for health care access and quality might justify the demand for private VHI by older people in Portugal.

2. Research design

2.1 Data and sample

We use data collected by the National Health Survey, which are representative of the Portuguese Population [34]. It is harmonized and regulated at the European level (EU regulation no 141/2013). It includes 18,204 individuals and our sample considers those aged over 65, that is, 5,701 individuals.

2.2 Variables

2.2.1 Dependent variable

The dependent variable is given by the question if the individual has voluntary health insurance. This is a binary variable that takes value 1 if the respondent has private health insurance and 0 otherwise.

2.2.2 Independent variables

Independent variables are grouped into five categories—demographic, socioeconomic, marital status, health status, related behavior, and insurance status. These variables are described in **Table 1**.

2.3 Quantitative analysis

The model to be estimated in this analysis is written as follows:

$$VHI_i{}^* = constant + \beta_i X_i + \varepsilon_i \; and = \begin{cases} 1 \text{ if } VHI_i^* \geq 0 \\ 0 \text{ if } VHI_i^* < 0. \end{cases} \quad (1)$$

where VHI* is the latent dependent variable, VHI is the observable dependent variable, β_i's are the coefficients to be estimated, X_i's are the independent variables, and ε_i is the residual.

Group of variables	Independent variables	Description
Demographic	Male	Dummy variable. Takes value 1 is male, 0 otherwise
	Age	Ordinal variable. Age is grouped into 15 classes. The first class takes value 1 and comprises ages 15–19; the last class takes value 15 and includes people older than 85. The variable is taken as continuous.
Socio-economic	Education	Ordinal variable. Education is grouped into five levels of education. First level 0 is those without schooling; fifth and last level is 5 and includes people with a college education. The variable is taken as continuous.
	Income	Ordinal variable. Income is grouped into five classes that represent the quantile of net monthly income per equivalent adult. The first value of income corresponds to the first quantile of income. The variable is taken as continuous.
	Urban	Dummy variable. Takes value 1 if the area is densely inhabited, 0 otherwise.
	Rural	Dummy variable. Takes value 1 if the area is sparsely inhabited, 0 otherwise.
	Moderate urban	Reference category.
Marital status	Single	Dummy variable. Takes value 1 if person is single; 0 otherwise.
	Married	Dummy variable. Takes value 1 if person is married; 0 otherwise.
	Divorced	Dummy variable. Takes value 1 if person is divorced; 0 otherwise.
	Widow	Reference category.
Health status and related behavior	SAH	Ordinal variable. Measures self-assessed health and ranges 1–5, where 1 means "very bad" and 5 "very good" health. The variable is taken as continuous.
	Chronic diseases	Dummy variable. Takes value 1 if person suffers from at least one chronic disease; 0 otherwise.
	Smoking	Dummy variable. Takes value 1 if person smokes; 0 otherwise.
	BMI	Body Mass Index.
Insurance status	ADSE	Dummy variable. Takes value 1 if person is covered through ADSE insurance; 0 otherwise.
	SAMS	Dummy variable. Takes value 1 if person is covered through SAMS insurance; 0 otherwise.
	Other insurance	Dummy variable. Takes value 1 if person has another occupational-based health insurance on top of NHS; 0 otherwise.
	NHS	Reference category. This is the case where respondents do not hold any occupational-based health insurance.

Table 1.
Description of independent variables.

The dependent variable expresses whether the respondent has voluntary health insurance. The binary nature of this variable implies that the econometric method of estimation is a probit. The estimated coefficients provide the direction of the relation between independent and dependent variables. The computation of the marginal effects allows the comparison of the intensity of the estimated coefficients. The marginal effects provide information on how the probability of having VHI changes when there is a unit change in the independent variable.

The results are obtained using Stata 15 econometric software.

3. Results

3.1 Descriptive statistics

The sample comprises 5,701 respondents older than 65, of whom 85.4% are retired. Only 332 respondents say that they have private voluntary health insurance, the large majority (about 94%) do not. Most of them are not entitled to any other insurance coverage apart from the NHS, and only about 10% are covered by ADSE, the occupation-based insurance plan for public workers (**Table 2**).

The remaining descriptive statistics for the independent variables are also shown in **Table 2**. The majority of the people in the sample are women (*circa* 61%) and most of them are aged between 65 and 75. Portuguese older people have very low levels of education, with more than 80% having less than 6 years of schooling. They have very low levels of income, about 50% receive an income valued in the first and second quintile of per capita household income. A large share of the people in the sample live in rural areas (*circa* 43%), and most of them are married or used to be married.

Finally, regarding their health status, the majority of older Portuguese assess their health status below the median level and about 86% of them report suffering from at least one chronic disease.

Other descriptive statistics regarding the distribution of respondents with private health insurance across income, education, and self-assessed health are shown in **Table 3**. Considering those individuals who said they had private health insurance (332 people), their distribution across income shows that a larger share of respondents has a high-income level. The distribution of people with health insurance across levels of education has two peaks, one at 6 years of schooling and the other at 17 years of schooling. The distribution of the health status of people having an insurance policy shows that most people with health insurance report a health status better than fair.

To finish the description of the variables, we now report the correlation between health risk indicators. The pairwise correlation between SAH and suffering from chronic diseases is equal to −0.364 and between SAH and smoking it is equal to 0.107, both for a statistical significance of less than 0.001. The tetrachoric correlation between smoking and suffering from a chronic disease is equal to −0.257 for an identical statistically significant level. So, there is no strong correlation that could prevent the joint utilization of these variables in a regression analysis.

3.2 Model results

The results obtained with the estimation of the probit for having voluntary health insurance are presented in **Table 4**. The statistically significant coefficients at 5% are marked with *.

The estimated coefficients show that as someone gets old or is single, the probability of having private health insurance decreases, while for higher income or education levels that probability increases.

Group of variables	Independent variables	Descriptive statistics	
		Number	%
Demographic	Male		
	Male	2,215	38.85
	Female	3,486	61.15
	Age		
	65–69	1,533	26.89
	70–74	1,319	23.14
	75–79	1,259	22.08
	80–84	979	17.17
	+85	611	10.72
Socio-economic status	Education (years)		
	0	1,942	34.06
	6	2,938	51.53
	9	353	6.19
	12	189	3.32
	15	14	0.25
	17	265	4.65
	Income (quantile)		
	Q1	1,368	24.00
	Q2	1.534	26.91
	Q3	1.174	20.59
	Q4	867	15.21
	Q5	758	13.30
	Level of urbanization		
	Urban	1,563	27.42
	Median	1,689	29.63
	Rural	2,449	42.96
	Retired		
	Yes	4,869	85.4
	Other status	832	14.6
Marital status	Marital status		
	Single	363	6.37
	Married	2,913	51.10
	Widow(er)	2,132	37.40
	Divorce	293	5.14
Health status and related behavior	SAH		
	1. Very bad	542	9.51
	2. Bad	1,443	25.33

Group of variables	Independent variables	Descriptive statistics	
		Number	%
	3. Fair	2,817	49.45
	4. Good	787	13.81
	5. Very good	108	1.90
	Chronic diseases		
	None	778	13.65
	At least one	4,992	86.35
	Smoker		
	Yes	266	4.7
	No	5,433	95.3
	BMI		
	Average	27.0	
Insurance status	Insurance		
	None (only NHS)	4,836	84.83
	ADSE	566	9.93
	SAMS	83	1.46
	Other insurance	216	3.78

Table 2.
Descriptive statistics.

Income						
Quantile	Q1	Q2	Q3	Q4	Q5	
number	21	31	50	66	164	
%	6.3	9.3	15.1	19.9	49.4	
Education						
years	0	6	9	12	15	17
number	30	120	63	42	3	74
%	9.1	36.1	19.0	12.7	0.0	22.3
SAH						
levels	1	2	3	4	5	
number	10	43	172	90	17	
%	3.0	13.0	51.8	27.1	5.1	

Table 3.
Distribution of respondents with voluntary health insurance.

Regarding the insurance status of people, being a beneficiary of ADSE or another occupation-based insurance decreases the odds of having private VHI. Lastly, the results for health status and health-related behavior are mixed. On the one hand, higher levels of SAH may be related to having VHI, but on the other hand, suffering from a chronic disease is also positively related to having VHI;

additionally, the observable behavior of smoking results in a lower likelihood of benefiting from VHI coverage.

The marginal effects associated with the most important and statistically significant coefficients are presented in **Table 5**.

These effects represent the change in the probability of having a VHI policy after the discrete change from the base level of the independent variable. In this way, the change to the oldest age groups implies a decrease of about 4% in the probability of having VHI, while the change from the lowest income quintile to the highest expresses an increase of 11% in the probability of being covered by VHI. Being a member of ADSE results in a 6% less chance of having VHI, and finally, the change from poor health status to a better one increases the likelihood of benefiting from a VHI; for instance, it increases almost 4% for people reporting very good health.

4. Discussion

In Europe, health systems tend to be mandatory and offer universal coverage. Despite this major trend, there is a market for voluntary private health insurance. Portugal is characterized by having a National Health Service of universal coverage with distinctive features of mandatory occupation-based insurance. Because the health insurance market suffers from asymmetric information, insurance companies adopt cream-skimming strategies to minimize adverse selection and moral hazards. One such strategy is to set the eligibility requirement for buying an insurance health policy is having to be under 65. In this way, most older people are unable to buy a health insurance policy. However, there is a small market and about 5% of Portuguese older people report having voluntary private health insurance of some kind.

Our aim in this work was to find the main determinants of the demand for private health insurance by older people in Portugal and contribute to the literature on voluntary health insurance schemes in different European countries, as there is no study for Portugal. We used data collected by the 2014 National Health Survey and estimated a probit for people over 65 having private health insurance.

The main results are aligned with previous studies concerning the importance of income and education [11, 16–19]. The higher the income and the better educated the individuals, the greater the probability of having private health insurance.

Concerning age and health insurance, we found that as they get older, they are less likely to have private voluntary health insurance [23, 35, 36]. The results show that only a minority of individuals, about 332 people, have a voluntary private health insurance policy. These people tend to have a high income and a high level of education, which is uncommon among people older than 65. Most older people in Portugal receive small pensions and have a low level of formal education, which deters them from taking out health insurance. The lack of schooling is the origin of illiteracy, both financial and health-related, which precludes people from making wiser choices on how to make better use of their savings and reduce future out-of-pocket expenditures. One major concern relates to dental care and the (high) associated cost. This aspect of health care is usually neglected by older people because it is not covered by the NHS and because they do not have a complementary private health insurance policy to cover it [37, 38].

Regarding the role of health status and behavior in explaining the demand for private health insurance, our results are mixed. On the one hand, there is some evidence of advantageous selection because better health status and no smoking are

		Coef.	Std. Err.	P > z
Demographic	Male	0,061	0,068	0,370
	Age group			
	70–74	−0.132	0.077	0.085
	75–79	−0.226*	0.089	0.011
	80–84	−0.497*	0.120	0.000
	+85	−0.469*	0.148	0.002
Socio-Economic	Education	0.073*	0.009	0.000
	Income			
	Q2	0.051	0.121	0.672
	Q3	0.353*	0.116	0.002
	Q4	0.542*	0.117	0.000
	Q5	0.988*	0.122	0.000
	Urban	0.112	0.077	0.146
	Rural	0.042	0.077	0.588
	Retired	−0.073	0.087	0.399
Marital status	Single	−0.367*	0.181	0.043
	Married	−0.039	0.118	0.738
	Widow(er)	−0.193	0.131	0.141
Insurance	ADSE	−0.647*	0.108	0.000
	SAMS	−0.200	0.179	0.265
	Other insurance	−0.410*	0.149	0.006
Health status and health behavior	SAH			
	2	0.128	0.160	0.424
	3	0.212	0.150	0.159
	4	0.330*	0.164	0.044
	5	0.392	0.226	0.083
	Chronic diseases	0.180*	0.091	0.047
	BMI	−0.006	0.008	0.405
	Smoking	−0.277*	0.135	0.041
	_cons	−2.285	0.318	0.000
	Number of obs	5,509		
	LR chi2(26)	518.92		
	Prob > chi2	0.000		
	Pseudo R2	0.207		
	Log likelihood	−994.916		

*Note: * Significant at less than 5%.*

Table 4.
Probit results.

	dy/dx	Std.Err.	P > z
Age group			
70–74	−0.015	0.008	0.083
75–79	−0.024	0.009	0.009
80–84	−0.044	0.009	0.000
+85	−0.042	0.011	0.000
Income			
Q2	0.003	0.006	0.670
Q3	0.025	0.008	0.002
Q4	0.045	0.010	0.000
Q5	0.117	0.016	0.000
Education	0.007	0.001	0.000
ADSE	−0.063	0.011	0.000
SAMS	−0.019	0.017	0.265
SAH			
2	0.010	0.012	0.402
3	0.018	0.011	0.112
4	0.030	0.014	0.026
5	0.038	0.024	0.109
Chronic diseases	0.017	0.009	0.047
Smoking	−0.027	0.013	0.041

Table 5.
Marginal effects.

associated with taking out health insurance. On the other, reported suffering from chronic diseases is also associated with health insurance, this time reflecting adverse selection.

It could be that insurance companies are discriminating based on observable traits, such as smoking. Or, related to high health risks, such as suffering from a chronic disease, it may be the case that people fail to report them. Perhaps insurance companies do not "cream skim" based on these conditions, either because they lack sufficient reliable information, or because they may calculate the probability that a person suffers from a certain disease at a certain age, or even because the insurance company can control claims associated with those health conditions by cost-sharing.

Another explanation of the mixed results found when relating health risk to health insurance is based on the demand side of the market. Maybe there is heterogeneity in the risk preferences of older people. In some countries, healthier individuals might be more risk-averse [14, 16] and so they are more prone to take out voluntary health insurance. Maybe this is the case with Portugal as it was with the UK [39]. On the other hand, people suffering from chronic diseases have a default health status that they consider to be a reference status in the sense proposed by the prospect theory [40]. These people may thus tend to be risk-averse with reference to their health status, and consequently, they are also more prone to have a private health insurance policy.

Finally, regarding the existence of parallel occupation-based insurance plans, our results indicate that people benefiting from ADSE, the largest occupation-based insurance for public servants, or from any other form of private or public health insurance (public health insurance is for the armed forces; private insurance includes bank workers, Portugal – Telecom workers, and postal CTT workers) are less likely to have VHI. This is expected to happen because occupation-based insurances provide a second layer of health coverage on top of the universal provided by the NHS. People benefiting from occupation-based insurance policies pay taxes to finance the NHS and pay a percentage of their income to finance occupation-based insurance. Therefore, this double financing by people deters them from looking for additional private health insurance coverage. In fact, these people do not need private health insurance because their health care needs are covered either by the NHS or by their occupation-based insurance.

The organization of the Portuguese health system creates inequity in access to health care. In the first place, people with double coverage have easier access to health care, and then people with high incomes can afford to buy private health insurance coverage. On top of this, inequality is aggravated by a tax system that gives some benefits to wealthier people for buying private health insurance or for spending on private health care [1]. The findings reported in this work confirm the existence of this sort of inequality, especially among older people.

One limitation of this work is that it is not possible to analyze the type of coverage provided to older people by voluntary private health insurance. This sort of information would show us what health care services older people want, and what could be lacking in the supply of NHS.

The results found in our analysis provide some insights into what makes older people decide to take out voluntary private health insurance. We have concluded that income is a determinant factor for taking out private health insurance, but it is also a factor for generating inequality in health care access. Older people can find it hard to access dental care or simple eye care because it is not covered by the NHS, or because the NHS waiting lists are too long. But the difficulty of complementing NHS coverage with private health insurance increases health care access inequity. Health and social policies may aim to narrow the gap either by providing health care in the NHS or by subsidizing the purchase of private health insurance for low-income older people. The first approach to this has already been put into place. The instrument called "dentist-check" for older people, created by the Ministry of Health attempts to mitigate the inequality in access to dental care, but it needs to be assessed.

Highlights

- small share of older people buy voluntary private health insurance
- higher income and higher education increase the likelihood of holding voluntary private health insurance
- benefiting from occupation-based insurance schemes reduce that likelihood
- voluntary private health insurance reflects inequity in healthcare access

Author funding

The author received no financial support for the research, authorship, and/or publication of this article.

Conflict of interest

The author declares no conflict of interest.

Declaration

The author declares this work does not require any human/animal subjects to acquire ethical approval.

JEL classification

I13; D81; C3

Author details

Aida Isabel Tavares[1,2]

1 ISEG, Lisbon School of Economics and Management, Lisbon, Portugal

2 CEISUC, Centre of Studies and Research in Health of the University of Coimbra, Coimbra, Portugal

*Address all correspondence to: atavares@iseg.ulisboa.pt

References

[1] Mossialos E, Thompson S. Report prepared for the Directorate General for Employment and Social Affairs of the European Commission. Brussels: European Commission; 2002

[2] Eurostat. Eurostat Database. 2020. Available from: https://ec.europa.eu/eurostat/data/database [Assessed: March 4, 2020]

[3] Simoes J, Augusto GF, Fronteira I, Hernández-Quevedo C. Portugal: Health system review. Health Systems in Transition. 2017;**19**(2):1-184

[4] Arrow K. Uncertainty and the welfare economics of medical care. The American Economic Review. 1963;**53**(5):941-973

[5] Rothchild M, Stiglitz J. Equilibrium in competitive insurance markets: An essay on the economics of imperfect information. Quarterly Journal of Economics. 1976;**90**(4):629-649

[6] Pauly MV. The economics of moral hazard: Comment. The American Economic Review. 1968;**58**(3):531-537

[7] Akerlof GA. The market for lemons: Quality uncertainty and the market mechanism. QJ Econ. 1970;**84**(3):488-500

[8] Hemenway D. Propitious selection. QJ Economics. 1990;**105**(4):1063-1069

[9] Einav L, Finkelstein A, Levin J. Selection in insurance markets: Theory and empirics in pictures. The Journal of Economic Perspectives. 2011;**25**(1):115-138

[10] Fang H, Keane M, Silverman D. Sources of Advantageous Selection: Evidence from the Meidgap Insurance Market. NBER Working Paper No. 12289; 2006

[11] Bolhaar J, Lindeboom M, van der Klaauw B. A dynamic analysis of the demand for health insurance and health care. European Economic Review. 2012;**56**(4):669-690

[12] Jones AM, Koolman X, Van Doorslaer E. The impact of having supplementary private health insurance on the use of specialists. Annales d'Economie et Statistique. 2006;**83**(84):251-275

[13] Paccagnella O, Rebba V, Weber G. Voluntary private health insurance among the over 50s in Europe. Health Economics. 2012;**22**(3):289-315

[14] Corea F. Big data and insurance: Advantageous selection in European Markets. Data Science Journal. 2017;**16**(33):1-15

[15] Outreville JF. Risk aversion, risk behavior, and demand for insurance: A survey. Journal of Insurance Issues. 2014;**37**(4):158-186

[16] Kiil A. What characterises the privately insured in universal health care system? A review of the empirical evidence. Health Policy. 2012;**106**:60-75

[17] Sliwinski A, Borkowska I. Private Voluntary Health Insurance: Market in Poland and Determinants of Demand—Review of Literature. In: Janowicz-Lomott M, Lyskawa K, Plychronidou P, Karasavvoglou A, editors. Economic and Financial Challenges for Balkan and Eastern European Countries. Switzerland: Springer; 2020

[18] Bolin K, Hedblom D, Lindgren A, Lindgren B. Asymmetric information and the demand for voluntary health insurance in Europe. NBER Working Paper. 2010:15689

[19] Tavares AI. Voluntary private health insurance demand determinants and risk preferences: Evidence from SHARE. The International Journal of Health Planning and Management. 2019;**2019**:1-19

[20] Oliveira M. Voluntary Health Insurance in Portugal: A Study for the European Commission. London: London School of Economics and Political Science; 2001

[21] Propper C, Rees H, Green K. The demand for private medical insurance in the UK: A cohort analysis. The Econometrics Journal. 2001;**111**(471):180-200

[22] Wagstaff A, van Doorslaer E. Measuring inequalities in health in the presence of multiple-category morbidity indicators. Health Economics. 1994;**3**:281-289

[23] Doiron D, Jones G, Savage E. Healthy, wealthy and insured? The role of self-assessed health in the demand for private health insurance. Health Economics. 2008;**17**(3):317-334

[24] Jofre-Bonet M. Public health care and private insurance demand: The waiting time as a link. Health Care Management Science. 2000;**3**:51-71

[25] Johar M, Jones G, Keane M, Savage E, Stavrunova O. Waiting times and the decision to buy private health insurance. Working Paper 2010/9. Centre for Health Economics Research and Evaluation, University of Technology Sydney; 2010

[26] De Meza D, Webb DC. Advantageous selection in insurance markets. The Rand Journal of Economics. 2001;**32**(2):249-262

[27] Buchmueller TC, Couffinhal A, Grignon M, Perronnin M. Access to physician services: Does supplemental insurance matter? Evidence from France. Health Economics. 2004;**13**(7):669-687

[28] Harmon C, Nolan B. Health insurance and health services utilization in Ireland. Health Economics. 2001;**10**(2):135-145

[29] Schokkaert E, van Ourti T, de Graeve D, Lecluyse A, van de Voorde C. Supplemental health insurance and equality of access in Belgium. Health Economics. 2010;**19**:377-395

[30] King D, Mossialos E. The determinants of private medical insurance prevalence in England, 1997-2001. Health Services Research. 2005;**40**(1):195-212

[31] Costa J, Garcia J. Demand for private health insurance: How important is the quality gap? Health Economics. 2003;**12**:587-599

[32] Saliba B, Ventelou B. Complementary health insurance in France. Who pays? Why? Who will suffer from public disengagement? Health Policy. 2007;**81**:166-182

[33] Jerant A, Fiscella K, Franks P. Health characteristics associated with gaining and losing private and public health insurance: A national study. Medical Care. 2012;**50**(2):145-151

[34] INE. National Health Survey. General information. 2014. Available from: https://www.ine.pt/xportal/xmain?xpid=INE&xpgid=ine_publicacoes&PUBLICACOESpub_boui=263714091&PUBLICACOESmodo=2&xlang=pt [Assessed: January 4, 2020]

[35] Emmerson C et al. Should private medical insurance be subsidised? Health Care UK. 2001:49-65

[36] Van De Ven W, Van Praag B. The demand for deductibles in private health insurance. Journal of Econometrics. 1981;**17**:229-252

[37] Carvalho C, Manso AC, Escoval A, Salvado F, Nunes C. Self-perception of oral health in older adults from an urban population in Lisbon, Portugal. Revista de Saúde Pública. 2016;**50**:50-53

[38] Kossioni AE. Is Europe prepared to meet the oral health needs of older people? Gerodontology. 2011;**29**(2):e1230-e1240

[39] Propper C. Constrained choice sets in the UK demand for private medical insurance. Journal of Public Economics. 1993;**51**:287-307

[40] Kahneman D, Tversky A. Prospect theory: An analysis of decision under risk. Econometrica. 1979;**47**:263-291

Chapter 8

Health Insurance in the United States: Failure of Private and Multi-Payer Financing

John Geyman

Abstract

Since the 1960s, the United States has subscribed to a business model of health care, largely for-profit with most private insurers on a mission to maximize their own revenues. Most insurers use cost sharing through deductibles and copayments based on the principle that enrollees will overuse health care services unless they have enough "skin in the game." As health care has been corporatized within a medical-industrial complex, even public insurers such as Medicare and Medicaid have been privatized with the same mission. Employer-sponsored health insurance has been the core of insurance in the U.S. since World War II, but has become unaffordable for employers and employees alike. This article brings historical perspective to how health insurance has been transformed from its not-for-profit origins in the 1930s, how it has become unaffordable in recent decades as it costs more and covers less, and how our multi-payer financing system has failed the public interest. Reform alternatives are discussed, but a system of universal coverage through a public, single-payer national plan is still beyond reach politically.

Keywords: health insurance, cost sharing, health care costs, cost containment, moral hazard, access to care, single payer financing, multi-payer financing, privatization, overpayments, Medicare, Medicaid, Medicare for all

1. Introduction

This is the U.S. story—from the birth of health insurance responding to genuine human need in the depths of the Great Depression in the 1930s—to the opulence of a massive corporatized industry today exploiting that need all the way to the bank. How do we explain that turn-around? This chapter has four goals: (1) to bring some historical perspective to that question; (2) to briefly summarize how health care services are bought and paid for in the U.S.; (3) to describe how private health insurance and multi-payer financing have failed the public interest; and (4) to compare four reform alternatives currently under consideration, only one of which will bring lasting reform through universal coverage.

2. Historical overview

Some in the U.S. considered the possibility of compulsory health insurance early in the 20th century after noting that 10 European countries had adopted one or another form of it by 1913 [1]. But that idea was controversial, and the emergence of voluntary, private health insurance in this country is especially attributed to a Blue Cross plan for school teachers in Dallas, Texas, in 1929. At that time as the Great Depression took hold, the nation's hospitals were in dire straits with more than one-third of the general hospital beds empty [2].

As the prototype upon which later Blue Cross plans were based, the Baylor plan provided free hospitalization for up to 21 days as well as coverage for operating room, laboratory and anesthesia services. The hospital assumed financial risk for hospital care without any third party and collected pre-payments. Other prepaid health insurance plans were soon to follow. The World War II years saw the start of employer-sponsored health insurance, when employers found it helpful to offer health insurance in order to recruit workers during a wartime economy with a severe labor shortage. By 1950, more than one-half of Americans were covered for the first time [3].

In the last 60-plus years, the private health insurance industry has been transformed from the quasi private-public partnership of its pioneering years to a massive industry on a corporate mission of profit over service. It has followed a conventional theory of insurance based on the concept of "moral hazard," whereby those with insurance are expected to overuse health care services and lead to uncontrolled increases in health care costs. As a result, community rating and guaranteed coverage during earlier years gave way to experience rating as medical underwriting became the new norm. The Blues were under pressure to compromise their earlier service mission, so that one-half of the nation's Blue Cross Blue Shield plans had consolidated and converted into for-profit companies by 2005 [4].

With some 1300 private insurers, the risk pool has fragmented into ever smaller parts as insurers work to avoid adverse selection. Medicare and Medicaid were enacted in 1965 as public plans, but recent decades have seen their increasing privatization that often ends up leaving many enrollees uninsured.

These are some of the many ways that insurers have used to extract more income at the expense of reliable and affordable coverage for enrollees:

2.1 Growth of a denial industry

"Denial management" became a growth industry of its own aimed at denying physicians' and hospitals' claims for services provided [5]. Many insurers developed ways of avoiding coverage of higher risk people in the first place. One such technique was to hold marketing meetings on the second floor of buildings without elevators to discourage less mobile and older people. Another technique was to make steep increases in premiums after receiving claims from enrollees who were sicker than expected. Denial of claims through burdensome pre-authorization of service became still another way to avoid paying expensive claims, increasingly associated with ever-changing networks. Out-of-network claims for hospital and physicians' services became unaffordable for many enrollees; even for in-network claims, the average denial rate today is 18% [6].

2.2 Managed care

Managed care grew rapidly during and after the 1990s, as a way to contain health care costs by changing from fee-for-service payment to prospective payment based upon capitation—the number of individuals enrolled in a health maintenance organization (HMO) plan. That gave insurers yet another way to profit from providing less care, and soon became known as managed *reimbursement* rather than managed care. As insurers found new profits, however, the quality and outcomes of care suffered. By 2000, 65 million Americans were enrolled in HMOs [7].

2.3 Privatization of public programs

Insurers have increasingly privatized Medicare and Medicaid in recent years as ways to exploit federal funding sources. Their claims that privatization would be more efficient have been proven false by experience. Instead, they have been more restrictive in choice and coverage, increased their administrative overhead to five or six times higher than traditional Medicare, and left markets that were insufficiently profitable. They have also increased their revenues by up-coding diagnoses—claiming payment for conditions for which care was not provided [8]. **Table 1** shows marked differences between privatized Medicare and traditional public Medicare by the early 2000s [9].

2.4 Consolidation and growing market power

Increasing consolidation through mergers within the private health insurance industry has taken place since the 1990s. The largest insurers today—in numeric order United Health Group, Anthem, Aetna and Cigna—collectively have a market share of 49% [10]. As a result, that level of consolidation has led to less competition, more cost sharing with higher deductibles, and less options for enrollees. United Health Group,

Privatized medicare	Original medicare
Experience-rated eligibility	Universal coverage
Managed competition	Social insurance as earned right
Defined contribution	Defined benefits
Segmented risk pool	Broad risk pool
Market pricing to risk	Administered prices
More volatile access & benefits	More reliable access & benefits
Increased cost sharing	Less cost sharing
Less accountability	Potential for more accountability
Less choice of provider & hospital	Full choice of provider & hospital
Less well distributed	Well distributed
Less efficiency, higher overhead	More efficiency, lower overhead

Source: Geyman [9].

Table 1.
Comparative features of privatized and public medicare (CAF Table 1.2, p. 14).

as the largest insurer in the country, has also gained clout beyond insurance by selling technology to hospitals, managing clinical trials, distributing prescription drugs, and offering continuing medical education to physicians [11].

3. How health care is paid for in the U.S.

Before looking at the role of private health insurance in U.S. health care, it is helpful (though still confusing!) to ask who really pays for health care. The late Dr. Uwe Reinhardt, Professor of Political Economy at Princeton University and author of *Priced Out: The Economic and Ethical Costs of American Health Care*, has summarized the complex transactions between enrollees in private households and providers of care in **Figure 1**. He makes the case that all health care spending originates from private households by paying premiums into public or private insurance pools as well as through taxes. The government accounts for about two-thirds of health care spending through taxpayer funding [12].

Today's system of paying for health care works against most of the working population through what economists call "labor income"—what people earn in their everyday jobs— that is taxed higher than "capital income" (accumulated wealth). As a result, billionaires today pay lower tax rates than their secretaries, steel workers, school teachers, and retirees [13].

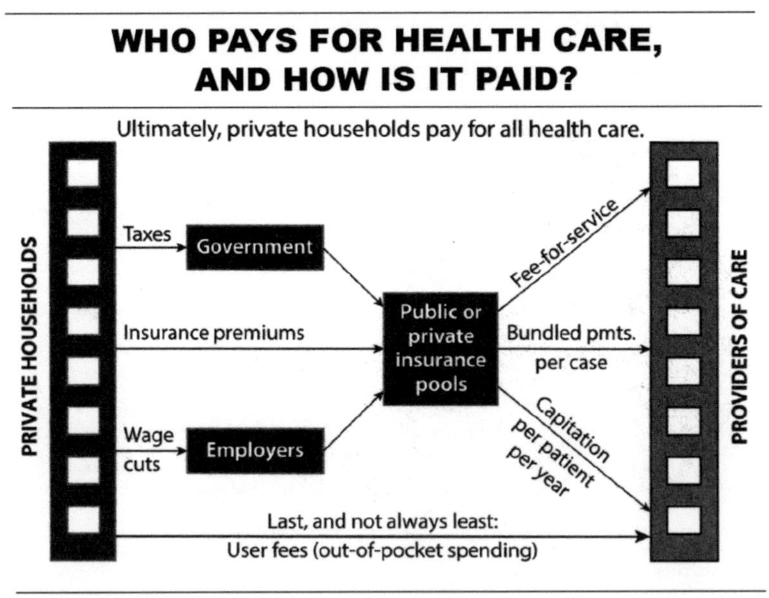

Figure 1.
Who pays for health care, and how is it paid (Figure 9.6, CAF 128).

4. How private health insurance and multi-payer financing have failed the public interest

These are some of the ways in which private health insurance and multi-payer financing have failed the common good in this country.

4.1 Unaffordable costs and increased cost sharing

Our market-driven system, now consolidated to a small number of corporate giants, can charge what the market will bear. Predictably, the cost of medical care has doubled compared to the consumer-price index over the last 25 years [14]. **Figure 2** shows the cumulative growth of the cost of premiums for employer-sponsored health insurance compared to annual average earnings of the bottom 90% over the last 20 years [15]. As a result, four in ten people with that insurance do not have enough savings to cover the deductibles and one in six have to cut back on food, take an extra job, or move in with friends or family [16]. Even when insured, many enrollees defer or avoid needed care, while many others receive high surprise medical bills that drag them into poverty, often ending them up in medical bankruptcy [17].

Predictably, increased cost sharing cuts access to care ranging from ER visits and office visits to hospital care and mental health [18]. As Dr. Veena Shankaran of the Hutchinson Cancer Research Center observes:

> *High-deductible plans are really the epitome of the access to care problem. People do not have the liquid cash to meet the deductible, so you see delays in care or even avoiding treatment altogether [19].*

4.2 Inadequate benefits

Private insurers have many ways to game the system at the expense of patients and taxpayers. Even after passage of the Affordable Care Act (ACA) in 2010, they discriminate against the sick by such benefit designs that limit access, high cost-sharing, restrictive drug formularies, inadequate and ever-changing networks of physicians and hospitals, and deceptive marketing practices. Meanwhile, they market new kinds of inadequate gap insurance, immune from the ACA's requirements, that include, for example, copays for treatment and lump sum payments upon diagnosis of such conditions as cancer, heart disease and stroke [20]. Short-term plans are another way

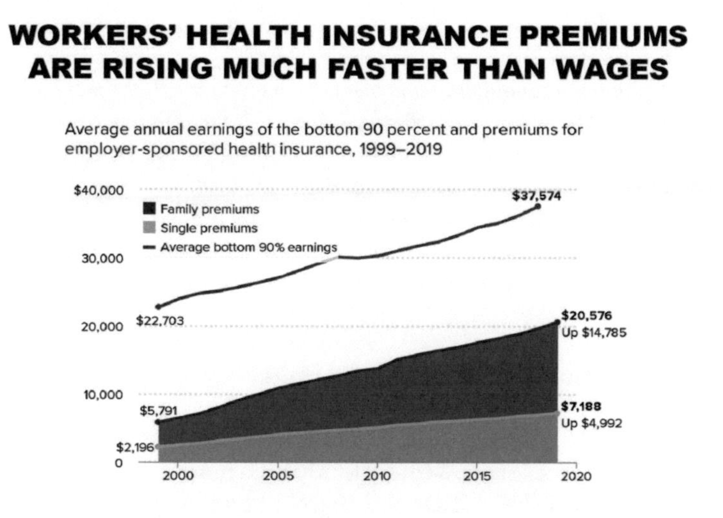

Figure 2.
(Figure 7.2 MIC 104).

to evade the ACA's requirements, providing very limited coverage for up to 1 year at exorbitant costs. Correctly labeled as "junk insurance," the aptly named Golden Rule Insurance has brought big profits to its owner, the giant United Health Group [21].

4.3 Profiteering

Private insurers consume 15–20% of the health care dollar in bureaucracy, administrative overhead, and profits. **Figure 3** shows how much higher that overhead is compared to other countries [22]. At the same time, they have received large subsidies from the federal government for many years, now about $685 billion a year [23] and projected by the Congressional Budget Office to double in another 10 years [24].

Overpayments for privatized Medicare and Medicaid have been a bonanza for private insurers, accounting for more than one-half of their net revenue. Their fraudulent practice of up-coding, mentioned above, accounts for much of that revenue, as shown in **Figure 4** [25].

Wall Street investors have much to say about what private insurers do in their unending quest for more profits. As one example, CVS Health, the parent company of Aetna, made far more money in 2021 than most other publicly traded corporations, in part because of Aetna's jacking up premiums and cost sharing, which it will do again in 2022. When the company issued a guidance for 2022 profits of just $12 billion to $13 billion (down just slightly from that for 2021 of $12.5 to $13 billion), its share price dropped by 6%, unnerving investors, and the company proceeded to buy back its own shares to boost earnings per share. Aetna's health insurance market has going down due to the decline of employer-sponsored health insurance, with less than one-third of businesses with 50 or fewer employees now offering health benefits [26].

Stepping back to consider all of this, Gerald Friedman, PhD, Professor of Economics at the University of Massachusetts Amherst and author of *The Case for Medicare for All*, brings us this important insight:

> *In many commodity markets, profits are a reward for making good products at low cost. Profits reward the company that makes the laptop, for example, giving it an incentive to produce a computer at low price; the more they sell, the more they profit. The incentives in health care are different, however. Rather than increasing sales, health insurers profit by screening customers, segmenting the market so as to exclude those likely to use health care ("lemon dropping") while attracting the healthy and lucky who use less health care (cherry picking"). While profitable, such activities add to the cost of America's bloated health care administration, raising a question that we should ask of all health care insurers: how many patients did your company help today? [27]*

4.4 Unreliability: exiting less profitable markets

Despite receiving long-term subsidies from the federal government, private health insurers leave their market, often with little advance notice, whenever their profits fall below expectations of their CEOs and shareholders. As just one example, at least 1.4 million people in 32 states lost their ACA coverage at the end of 2016, leaving them fewer choices than before [28].

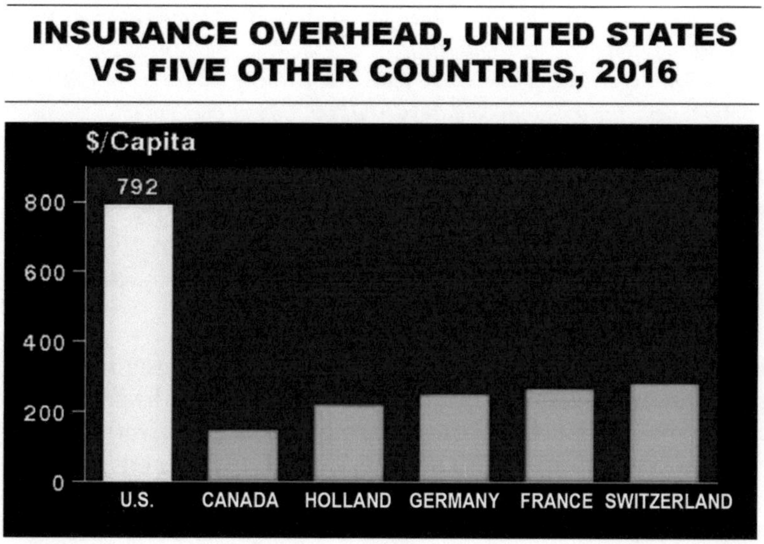

Figure 3.
Insurance overhead in 6 countries (CAF Figure 11.2, 151).

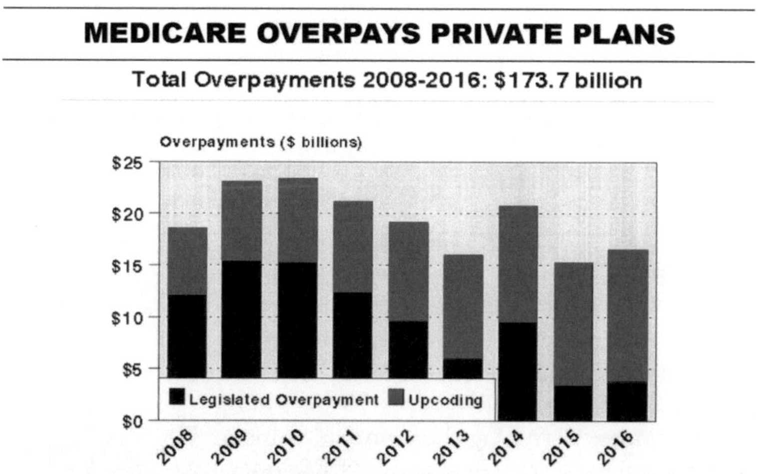

Figure 4.
(CAF Figure 4.2, 45)

4.5 Segmented risk pools

To be effective nationally, health insurance must be compulsory in order to eliminate segmentation of risk pools, as Dr. Henry Sigerist, then Director of the History of Medicine at the Johns Hopkins University, recognized as far back as 1944:

> *Illness is an unpredictable risk for the individual family, but we know fairly accurately how much illness a large group of people will have, how much medical care they will require, and how many days they will have to spend in hospitals. In other*

> *words, we cannot budget the cost of illness for the individual family but we can budget it for the nation. The principle must be to spread the risk among as many people as possible ... The experience of the last 15 years in the United States [since 1931] has, in my opinion, demonstrated that voluntary health insurance does not solve the problem of the nation. It reaches only certain groups and is always at the mercy of economic fluctuations ... Hence, if we decide to finance medical services through insurance, the insurance system must be compulsory [29].*

5. Reform alternatives

The above account of the expensive missteps in U.S. health insurance over these many years shows how important universal coverage is to meet the needs of our population, as has been shown in many advanced countries around the world. Remarkably, a proposal was made for national health insurance by Teddy Roosevelt as a presidential candidate on the progressive ticket more than a century ago in 1912. It was rejected then and thereafter as the political debate became controlled by corporate stakeholders in the present lucrative financing "system." With health care now accounting for more than one-sixth of the nation's GDP, corporate power and lobbying for its continuance have continued to block reform efforts for cost containment, health care equity, and universal coverage. It has become increasingly clear that employer-sponsored health insurance has itself been a big part of the problem, as Drs. Anne Case and Angus Deaton, Professors Emeritus of Economics and Public Affairs at Princeton University recently observed:

> *The historical accident of employer-based coverage is a huge barrier to reform. So is the way that the health care industry is protected in Washington by its lobbyists—five for every member of Congress [30].*

Health care has become a front-burner issue in recent political campaigns and as we head into the 2022 and 2024 election cycles. These four reform alternatives are up for debate:

1. Building on the Affordable Care Act (ACA) of 2010;

2. Medicare for Some: increasing the numbers of insured by Medicare by lowering the eligibility age to 60, together with a public option for sale alongside private plans on the ACA's exchanges;

3. Privatized Medicare Advantage for All; and

4. Single-payer Medicare for All.

The first three of these alternatives would leave a for-profit, multi-payer financing system in place with all of the problems described previously. The fourth alternative is the only one that can bring a not-for-profit public financing system with universal coverage for all Americans, cost containment, improved access and quality of care. There is a bill in the House of Representatives (H. R. 1976) for Medicare for All with more than 120 co-sponsors. However, the Congress is sharply divided along partisan lines, and this bill may have to wait for the forthcoming elections for the Congress to clarify its priorities.

Although much of organized medicine in the U.S. has opposed national health insurance over the years, that stance is beginning to change as so many physicians find our present multi-payer financing system such an impediment to daily medical practice. Medicare for All already has strong support among the general public, physicians and nurses. Experience and evidence over the years confirms its advantages as shown by **Table 2** [31]. Had Medicare for All been in place during 2019, it is estimated that we would have saved more than $1 trillion. **Figure 5** shows how those savings would have been taken place [32].

If and when Medicare for All can be enacted, it will bring a new system of national health insurance for all Americans with comprehensive benefits based on medical need, not ability to pay, together with full choice of hospitals, physicians and other health professionals anywhere in the country. Administrative simplification will drop its single-payer overhead to about 3%, one-sixth of today's multi-payer overhead.

	ACA	Public option	Medicare advantage for all	Medicare for all
Access	Restricted	Restricted	Restricted	Unrestricted
Choice	Restricted	Restricted	Restricted	Unrestricted
Cost containment	Never	Never	Never	Yes
Quality of care	Unacceptable	Unacceptable	Unacceptable	Improved
Bureaucracy	Large, wasteful	Large, wasteful	Large, wasteful	Much reduced
Universal coverage	Never	Never	Never	Yes
Accountability	No	No	No	Yes
Sustainability	No	No	No	Yes

Table 2.
Comparison of four reform alternatives based on evidence (Table 13.1, 60 years, 160).

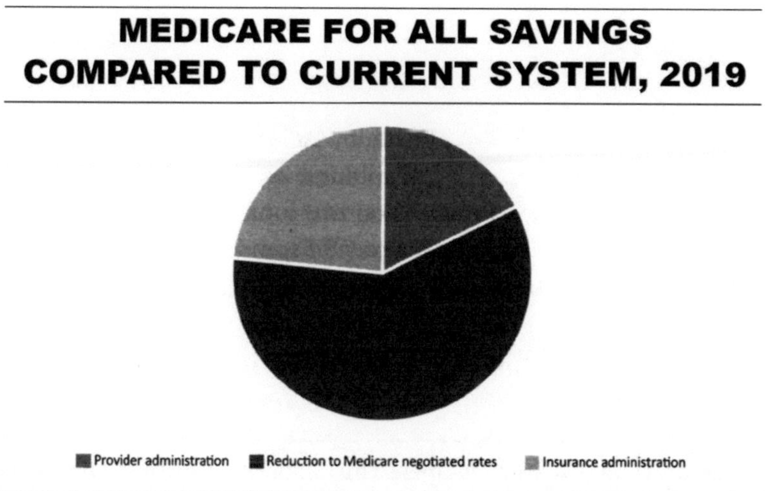

Figure 5.
Medicare for all savings compared to current system, 2019 (Figure 14.2, MIC 269).

Cost savings will be achieved through large-scale cost controls, including (a) negotiated fee schedules for physicians and other health professionals, who will remain in private practice; (b) global annual budgeting of hospitals and other facilities; and (c) bulk purchasing of drugs and medical devices. Cost sharing through deductibles and copayments will be eliminated at the point of service, and pre-authorization of services will no longer be needed. Higher priority will be given to primary care and public health, while the risk for costs of illness and accidents will be shared across our entire population of 330 million Americans.

6. Conclusion

The corporate transformation of health care in this country from a traditional service ethic to a commodity for sale in an unfettered marketplace is indeed unfortunate. Financing reform through a not-for-profit public mechanism—Medicare for All—can go a long way to restoring the traditional service ethic of health care as a moral enterprise. We shall see what the future will bring. Meanwhile, Winston Churchill gives us hope:

> *Americans will always do the right thing—after they exhaust all the alternatives.*

Author details

John Geyman
Family Medicine, University of Washington School of Medicine, Seattle, WA, USA

*Address all correspondence to: jgeyman@uw.edu

References

[1] Starr P. The Social Transformation of American Medicine. New York: Basic Books; 1982. pp. 252-253

[2] Stuart JE. The Blue Cross Story: An Informal Biography of the Voluntary Prepayment Plan for Hospital Care. Chicago: BCBSA Archives; 1966. p. 19

[3] Hacker JS. The Great Risk Shift: The Assault on American Jobs, Families, Health Care, and Retirement, and How You Can Fight Back. New York: Oxford University Press; 2006. p. 145

[4] Fuhrmans V. Billing battle. Fights over health claims spawn a new arms race. Wall Street Journal. 2007:A1

[5] Schramm C. The Diseconomies of Blue Cross Conversion. Washington, D.C.: Alliance for Advancing Non-Profit Health Care; 2005

[6] Silvers JB. This is the Most Realistic Path to Medicare for All. New York Times; 2019

[7] Jensen GA, Morrissey MA, Gaffney S, et al. The new dominance of managed care: Insurance trends in the 1990s. Health Affairs (Millwood). 1997;**16**(1):125-136

[8] Livingston S. Insurers profit from Medicare Advantage's incentive to add coding that boosts reimbursement. Modern Healthcare. 2018

[9] Geyman JP. Shredding the Social Contract: The Privatization of Medicare. Monroe, ME: Common Courage Press; 2006. p. 206

[10] Waddill K. Health insurance consolidation grew from 2014 to 2020. Health Payer Intelligence. 2021

[11] Murphy T. United Health Looks Beyond Insurance to Help Fuel 4Q Growth. New York City, New York: Associated Press; 2017

[12] Reinhardt UE. Priced Out: The Economic and Ethical Costs of American Health Care. Princeton, NJ: Princeton University Press; 2019. p. 63

[13] Saez E, Zucman G. The Triumph of Injustice: How the Rich Dodge Taxes and How to Make Them Pay. New York: W. W. Norton & Company; 2019. p. xi

[14] Gillers H. Retiree health benefits cut. Wall Street Journal. 2019

[15] KFF Health Affairs. Average Family Premiums Rose 4 Percent to $21,342 in 2020, Benchmark KFF Employer Health Benefit Survey Finds. KFF; 2020

[16] Levey NN. Health Insurance Deductibles Soar, Leaving Americans with Unaffordable Bills. Los Angeles Times; 2019

[17] Himmelstein DU, Lawless RM, Thorne D, et al. Medical bankruptcy: Still common despite the Affordable Care Act. American Journal of Public Health. 2019;**109**(3):431-433

[18] The Editors. Out of Pocket, out of control. Bloomberg View. 2015

[19] Shankaran V. As quoted by Stallings, E. High-deductible health policies linked to delayed diagnosis and treatment. NPR. 2019

[20] Silverman RE. For workers, an 'insurance on insurance.' Wall Street Journal. 2016:B5

[21] Hiltzic M. Why the Short-term Health Plans are Cheap: They

Shortchange you on Care. Los Angeles Times; 2019

[22] Organization for Economic Cooperation and Development. 2016

[23] Ockerman E. It Costs $685 Billion a Year to Subsidize U. S. Health Insurance. Bloomberg News; 2018

[24] Potter W. Take it from Me, Tweaks won't Fix Health Care. USA Today; 2018

[25] Geruso M, Layton T. Up-coding Inflates Medicare Costs in Excess of $2 Billion Annually. UT News, University of Texas at Austin; 2015

[26] Potter W. Despite a Profitable 2021, Expect Higher Deductibles and Premiums in Aetna's Health Plans for 2022. Wendell Potter NOW; 2022

[27] Friedman G. An Open Letter to the New York Times that was Rejected. 2016

[28] Tracer Z, Darie T. More than 1 Million in Obamacare to Lose Plans as Insurers Quit. Bloomberg News; 2016

[29] Sigerist H. Medical care for all the people. Canadian Journal of Public Health. 1944;**35**(7):258

[30] Case A, Deaton A. The Sickness of Our System. Time; 2020. p. 81

[31] Geyman JP. Transformation of U. S. Health Care: 1960-2020: One Family Physician's Journey. Friday Harbor, WA: Copernicus Healthcare; 2022. p. 160

[32] Freidman E. The Case for Medicare for All. Medford, MA: Polity Press; 2020. p. 62

Chapter 9

Value-Based Contracting in Health Care

Ian Duncan

Abstract

A growing topic in healthcare in the United States and other countries is the decentralization of risk from the ultimate healthcare payer (insurance companies and government in the United States; national health systems in other countries) to providers of healthcare services. Healthcare providers have traditionally taken clinical risk.[1] However, payers are increasingly looking to providers to assume financial risk, in addition to the risk of clinical quality and outcomes of their managed populations. Numerous different types of contracts are being signed between providers and payers: pay for quality; pay for performance; shared risk and shared savings arrangements; bundled payments, accountable care and capitation (full or partial risk). Any contracting entity must decide what is the right form of contract to enter, what contract features to include and what price to offer the payer and what risk the entity is assuming in doing so. The assessment of opportunity, design of the contract terms, pricing, risk management and outcomes evaluation for these contracts are increasingly complex exercises. This chapter covers these issues, including the actuarial mathematics of contract risk assessment and mitigation, taking the reader through the 5 components of a Value-based contract.

Keywords: financial risk, model accuracy, opportunity assessment, economic modeling

1. Introduction

At its most fundamental, health risk (either clinical or financial) is a combination of two factors: **amount of loss** and **probability of occurrence**. For the purpose of this chapter we define a loss as having occurred when an individual's post-occurrence state is less favorable than the pre-occurrence state. Financial Risk is a function of Loss Amount and Probability of Occurrence, or in actuarial terminology, frequency and severity of loss. In the United States health risk has historically been the responsibility of payers (insurers, government programs and employers). Healthcare payers have traditionally managed risk by a combination of pricing, underwriting, and reinsurance, together with claims management.

[1] Clinical risk represents the responsibility that clinicians assume for the health outcomes of their patients. This chapter covers financial risk, or the cost of care for patients.

With the enactment of the HMO Act of 1973 (42 U.S.C. § 300e), **Managed Care** developed in the 1990s as a series of initiatives designed to better manage the health of covered individuals and reduce unnecessary medical claims costs. The original approaches included **network management** (identifying and contracting with preferred providers who offered either lower fees or lower utilization of services and steering patients to them, either through benefit design or by requiring referrals) and **utilization management** (pre-authorization or concurrent review of hospital admissions). In a quest for savings these models devolved into restriction of services and denials of care. Because of consumer reaction to the perceived restrictions and denials that resulted from these interventions, managed care plans began to seek other solutions to contain rapidly increasing costs. Techniques that were favored for managing utilization include the implementation of programs that encourage members to take responsibility for their own health, or that aimed to educate physicians in the most cost-effective, evidence-based treatments (Chronic disease management and case management).

The chronic disease management (DM) programs of the early 2000s were implemented by payers and aimed to identify high risk or high need patients, particularly those that were not compliant with their treatments or who had gaps in care. Patient management was usually performed externally, often by telephone, by nurses employed by large disease management organizations. Although attempts were made to involve the patient's providers, providers were not party to the payer contract. This model reached its peak with a number of Medicare Coordinated Care and Support demonstration programs between 2005 and 2008 [1, 2]. Because of the growth and importance of chronic disease management programs, the Centers for Medicare and Medicaid Services (CMS) of the US Dept. of Health and Human Services (HHS) established a major demonstration project, the Medicare Coordinated Care Project to evaluate 15 different models of care coordination [2, 3]. Although the demonstration program showed some improvement in the quality of care delivered to patients, the lack of demonstrated savings led to a decline in the type of vendor-based disease management programs popular up to that time, and an interest in programs that involved contracting directly with providers to take risk for patient outcomes.

By the end of the first decade of the 21st Century two things began to become clear: first, that these programs were not containing medical trend[2] and second that the solution to rising costs had to include providers. As a result, CMS's attention shifted to alternative payment models incorporating providers directly and focusing on a combination of cost, quality and patient satisfaction, an objective expressed by Berwick and others [4] as the "Triple Aim" in a heavily cited article. This shift was a reaction to the quality of care delivered within the US Healthcare system. A 2003 study [5] found that adults in the United States receive the generally accepted standard of preventive, acute, and chronic care only about 55% of the time. Quality of care "varied substantially according to the particular medical condition, ranging from 78.7 percent of recommended care to 10.5 percent of recommended care for alcohol dependence." Pay for quality was intended increase the frequency of these

[2] "Healthcare Trend" (Trend) is defined as the proportional increase in the cost of care per member per month (PMPM). Trend is a combination of several factors, including medical inflation (increase in the cost of the basket of services); increased units of services consumed; increased intensity of services and enhanced technology.

measures by rewarding physicians for their achievement of evidence-based quality measures (such as screenings, tests for patient populations or adherence to prescriptions). The theory was that closing gaps in care and identifying health issues earlier would lead to reduced utilization of more expensive healthcare services later. The achievement of reduced cost of care in exchange for incentive payments made this a value-based initiative.

Following the failure of the disease management model to demonstrate financial success, Congress has passed a number of laws promoting different value-based initiatives, in addition to initiatives introduced by the Center for Innovation at CMS:

- Medicare Improvements for Patients and Providers Act (MIPPA) 2008;
- Affordable Care Act (ACA) 2010;
- Bundled Payments for Care Improvement (BPCI and its successors) 2011;
- Protecting Access to Medicare Act (PAMA) 2014;
- The Medicare Access and CHIP Reauthorization Act (MACRA) 2015;
- Medicare's direct contracting model: Global and Professional Direct Contracting Model (GPDC) 2020.

In addition, CMS has introduced a number of alternative payment models (APMs). In these models, providers agree to accept a portion of their reimbursement, often in the form of a share of savings, based on achievement of certain goals, including improved quality, reduced utilization and reduced cost. APMs include Accountable Care Organizations (ACOs) as well as models aimed at specific conditions or provider organizations: Bundled Payments for Care Improvement (BPCI), Comprehensive Care for Joint Replacement, Comprehensive Primary Care, Comprehensive End-stage Renal Disease model, Kidney Care Choices model, and the Oncology Care Model (OCM). CMS's stated objective is to move the entire health care market toward paying providers based on the quality, rather than the quantity of care they give patients.[3]

The Health Care Payment Learning and Action Network (HCP-LAN) is a group of public and private health care leaders launched by the U.S. Department of Health and Human Services (through CMS) in March 2015. HCP-LAN aligns public and private sector stakeholders in shifting away from the current fee-for-service, volume-based payment system to one that pays for high-quality care and improved health. HCP-LAN has published estimates of value-based contract penetration in different payer segments. **Figure 1** illustrates a study published in 2019 predicting that as much as 100% of care will be delivered via a value-based contract by 2025.

The HCP-LAN 2020 survey of payers indicated that 40.9% of U.S. health care payments, representing approximately 238.8 million Americans and 80.2% of the covered population, flowed through HCP-LAN Categories 3&4 models (shared-risk and population-based payments).

[3] https://www.cms.gov/Medicare/Quality-Initiatives-Patient-Assessment-Instruments/Value-Based-Programs/Value-Based-Programs.

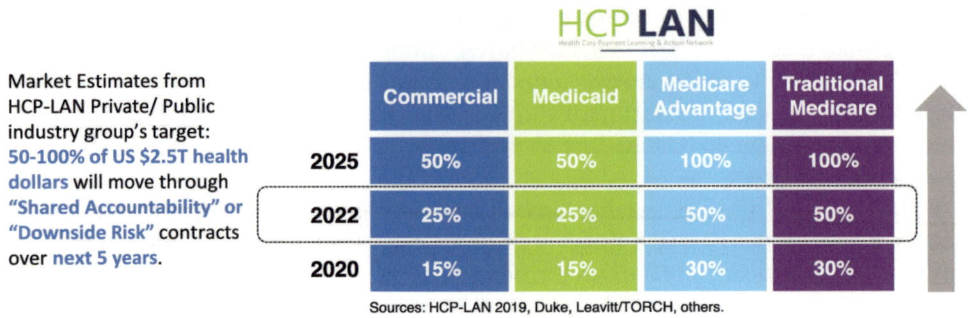

Figure 1.
Estimates of value-based contract growth in different payer segments.

2. Types of value-based contracts

As noted by Werner et al. in a 2021 study [6] "the complexity of the current suite of alternative payment models" and the variety and lack of standardization of different models make value-based contracting challenging. **Figure 2** illustrates the development and growth of alternative payment models over time. The following discussion of contract types covers a broad (but not necessarily exhaustive) spectrum: new variations are frequently introduced. Over time, models have become more comprehensive and the risk assumed by providers and healthcare management organizations (HCMs) has increased.

Figure 2 illustrates the two dimensions of risk that are accepted by a provider or HCM: the x-axis indicates increasing degrees of financial risk, from none (pay for performance or pay for quality which represent supplemental payments on top of regular provider reimbursement) to capitation (which represents the potential for significant gain but also losses). The y-axis illustrates the extent of the services at risk

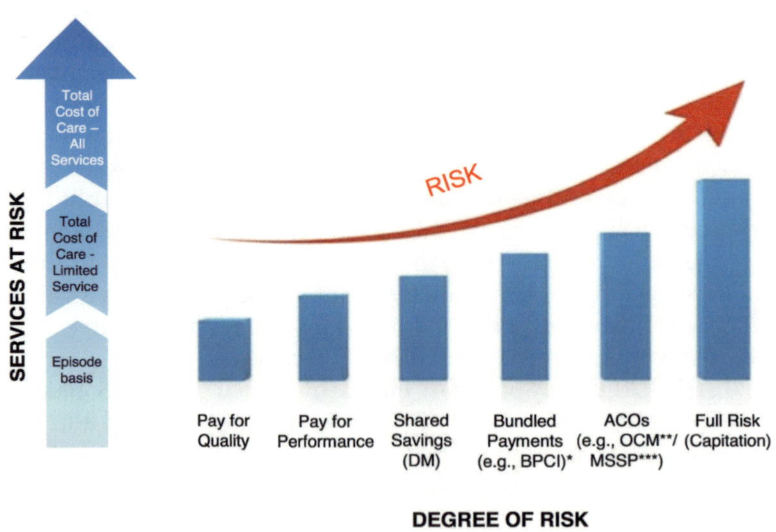

Figure 2.
*Risk and VBC contract types. *BPCI: Bundled Payment for Care Improvement; **OCM: Oncology Care Model; ***MSSP: Medicare Shared Savings Program.*

incorporated in the contract, which may range from a risk limited to a single episode of care only (for example knee surgery) to population risk. Population risk in turn may be limited to certain services only (for example for maternity services those associated with the pregnancy only) to "total cost of care" in which the provider or HCM accepts financial risk for all expenses incurred by the target population.

As we discussed above, the original reimbursement model was fee-for-service: each time the patient received a service from a physician, hospital or pharmacist a bill was generated and then paid by the patient or the payer (or both). As this system began to impose a financial strain on payers, different models evolved, beginning with payment for quality. Payment for quality models addressed the "gaps in care" issue identified in [5], as well as attempting to limit the provision of excess and ultimately redundant services. While these models resulted in improvement in quality metrics (such as HEDIS https://www.ncqa.org/hedis/) they did not lead to significant reduction in healthcare costs. Closely allied to pay for quality models is pay for performance in which physicians are rewarded for patient metrics (such as mammograms for women, eye and foot exams for people with diabetes, etc.).

The big breakthrough in terms of financial risk transfer occurred with disease management programs in the early 2000s. Insurers that purchased disease management programs from vendors needed assurance that the programs would reduce medical cost. Lacking convincing randomized studies, vendors and payers contracted around a financial outcome; initially vendors put a portion of their fees at risk of a favorable financial outcome. Later models allowed vendors to share in actual savings generated (gain-sharing), to the extent that the vendor reduced costs below a target. There are different variations of gain-sharing models, with some being one-sided (only positive savings are shared) while others are two-sided (if costs increase relative to the target, the vendor must reimburse some portion of the excess). More discussion of these models and methods for measuring financial outcomes may be found in Duncan [7].

CMS introduced another value-based arrangement with its Bundled Payment initiative in which organizations entered into payment arrangements that included financial and performance accountability for episodes of care. These models aimed to increase quality and care coordination at a lower cost to CMS. Providers continue to bill CMS in the usual way, with a retrospective reconciliation of claims against a previously agreed upon target price. Depending on which of four payment models the provider enters into, the provider receives a payment that covers hospital only or hospital plus physician services. To the extent that the provider is able to manage the financial risk, it keeps the financial margin (in some models the provider is responsible for reimbursing CMS if costs exceeded target prices). See [8] for a description of the different BPCI models and the results of evaluations.

The Affordable Care Act (2010) [9] introduced Accountable Care Organizations (ACOs): provider groups that accept payment risk for their attributed populations in return for the opportunity to share savings when costs are reduced below an adjusted benchmark. In the original model providers only accepted upside risk (shared savings only). In later models providers could achieve a greater share of savings but at the cost of having to share also in losses. More detail may be found in [10]. ACO arrangements exist among all payers and payer types, including commercial insurers, traditional Medicare and Medicaid. CMS's Oncology Care Model is a similar initiative but limited to cancer patients undergoing treatment by oncologists.

All these models involve some sharing of risk between the payer and providers. Full risk transfer is achieved with capitated models. With capitation the provider accepts full financial responsibility for all costs of a population (or sub-population, for example primary care only).

3. Five steps to value-based contracting

Value-based contracting requires a clinical organization that is different to the traditional practice management. Several texts discuss necessary re-organization of clinical practice and the necessary infrastructure [11–16] etc. For the purposes of this chapter we assume that clinical delivery has been optimized and the provider of clinical services is ready to begin the financial modeling required to negotiate contract with a payer.

We illustrate the contract modeling and implementation steps in **Figure 2**.

Successful value-based contracting requires sophisticated analytics, and at the heart of the analysis is a robust data warehouse that integrates claims data, preferably with clinical data. The importance of claims data is often overlooked by providers, with their focus on clinical data, charts and electronic medical records. Healthcare claims in the US system are the basis of reimbursement, containing valuable information about the nature and diagnosis of a patient's condition, the treatment applied by the physician or health system, the place of service and (in the case of drugs) the therapeutic class and dosage of a drug. Complete medical and drug claims—claims that include all providers utilized by a population—are essential for financial contracting but are seldom present in provider records: they must be obtained from a payer. Providers rarely have as complete a view of the patient's care that the payer has (due to its contracts with multiple providers).[4] Once a robust warehouse has been built, it is possible to begin the five steps to successful value-based contracting (**Figure 3**).

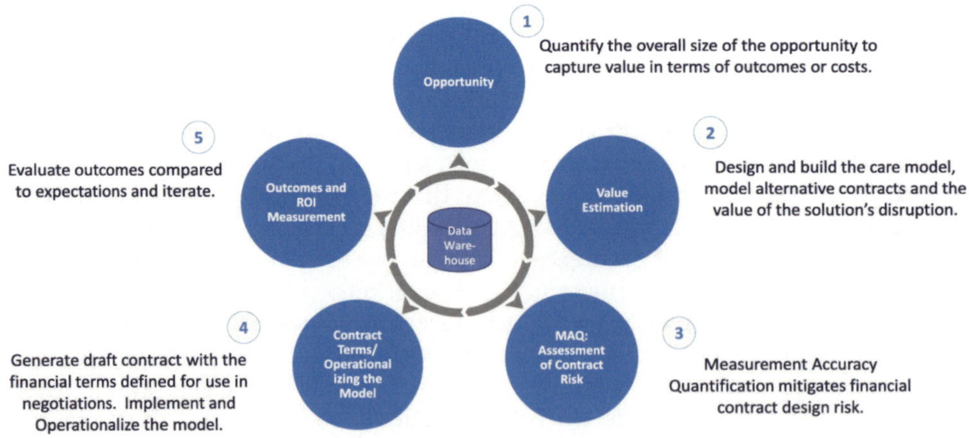

Figure 3.
Five steps to successful value-based contracting.

[4] For more detail about healthcare claims and the information they contain, see Chapter 3 of Ian Duncan: *Healthcare Risk Adjustment and Predictive Modeling 2nd edition*. 2018, New Hartford CT: Actex Publications.

3.1 Step 1: opportunity analysis

For any start-up or mature company wishing to enter a value-based contract, the essential first step is to assess the financial opportunity. Payers are subject to multiple new opportunities weekly; a provider or HCM must make a compelling economic case to gain attention. The compelling economic case begins with **opportunity.** Said differently, does what the provider or HCM intend to contract for address sufficient healthcare spending to be interesting to the payer? Opportunity analysis requires a detailed analysis of healthcare spending on the condition or procedure that the provider or HCM intends to manage. This type of analysis requires detailed healthcare spending (claims) data for the business segment in which the provider or HCM operates. Analysis should address condition prevalence and utilization of the targeted condition(s) and estimate the addressable cost they impose. To gain a payer's attention the provider/HCM must address an economic concern, which in turn combines two elements:

- Frequency: the condition or procedure must occur with sufficient frequency to be of concern to the payer.

- Severity: the cost imposed by the condition or procedure must be high enough to command the payer's attention.

Some conditions impose one but not the other of these elements: for example, in an employer population, an episode of stroke is very high cost but occurs with sufficiently low frequency that the average employer may not have experienced a recent stroke in its population. Employees that suffer strokes experience lengthy episodes, during which another payer (such as Social Security disability, or a retirement plan) may become responsible for reimbursement. As a result, the employer may not view strokes as a concern. Cancer, in the other hand, imposes high costs episodically but with cancer diagnoses occurring frequently enough for a payer to be concerned with managing cancer costs.

Modeling opportunity, particularly for individual diagnoses, requires access to large databases. These may be purchased from data vendors, or providers/HCMs may contract with a consultant for this phase of work.

3.2 Step 2: value estimation and economic modeling

Pricing a value-based contract requires an estimate of the value that will be created by a program, device or other intervention (in addition to estimates of the cost of delivery of the VBC solution). Value estimation requires identification of the patient's current treatment pathway and a projection of an alternative pathway once a VBC solution is implemented. The treatment pathway is a transition or multi-state model that identifies different branches that a patient can follow together with the probability and cost of each different branch. **Figure 4** is an example of a simple multi-state model of a specific condition for which the patient can choose to receive treatment in an urgent care setting or a hospital Emergency Department (ED). Depending on the severity of the condition, a patient in the urgent care setting could be sent home or referred to ED. A patient seeking care in the ED could be tested and sent home or, after referral for further evaluation, either sent home or admitted to hospital.

A detailed claims database will allow the analyst to assess the services, their frequency and the pathway that a typical patient follows. As **Figure 4** shows, we associate transition frequencies with the different states, as well as the cost of treatment

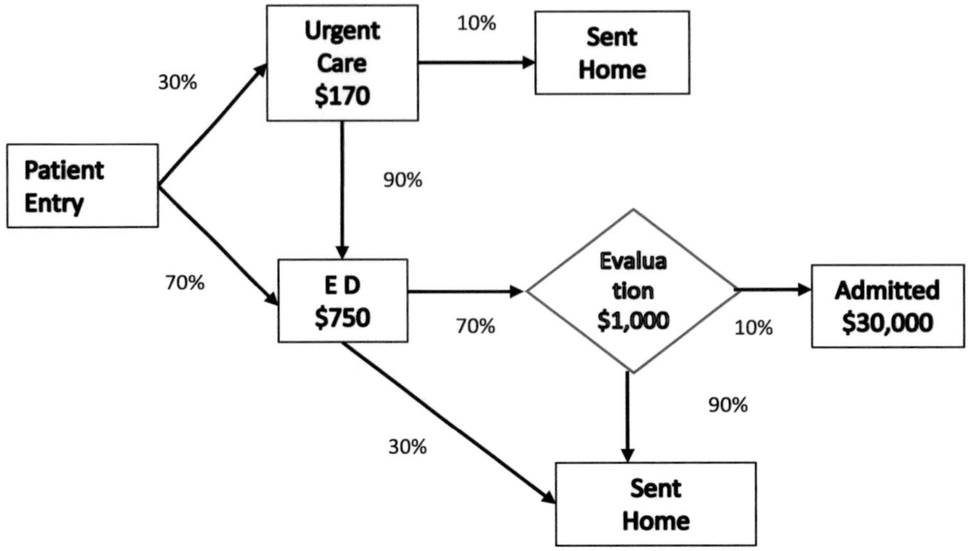

Figure 4.
Current patient pathway.

at different stages. A disruptive device or intervention in this model would reduce the frequency of transition to higher-cost pathways. **Figure 4** is a simple pathway; pathways can become extremely complex, in which case some simplification will be necessary. Complexity arises not because of the variety of settings but because the services that the patient receives may be delivered in a different order (for example for some cancer patients, oncology may be delivered first, followed by surgery while for other patients, surgery may be performed first, followed by oncology). Episodes of care that involve physician or auxiliary providers (for example physical therapy) may involve a few treatments over time, to as many as one or two per week.

Once the typical patient pathway is defined and its frequencies and costs have been developed, the analyst can develop an alternative pathway, assuming the provider/HCM intervention has been applied. The alternative pathway illustrates the disruption to the current standard of practice that the provider intervention generates; this may be estimated from prior studies or simply by clinicians who understand the intervention. The difference between the current and proposed pathways, however, is the source of the estimation of the provider's or HCM's economic value added. The result of this analysis is an economic model which is the basis of the HCM's pricing. The economic model is developed by comparing frequencies and unit costs under the current and proposed pathways.

Understanding pathways is a critically important component of the financial estimation process. Providers/HCMs often spend time and effort on the financial estimation phase and assume that the actual work of caring for patients and driving behavior change will take care of itself, if left to clinicians. Clinicians, however, need to know where and how they can perform interventions, with what patients and what outcome to expect. Operationalizing the model to achieve the projected savings is as important as understanding the opportunity. Pathway analysis can provide valuable input to this process because it provides a basis for breaking savings assumptions into drivers/components. We will return below to considering the implementation of a value-based contract.

Current patient pathway				**Proposed patient pathway**		
Setting	**Patients**	**Charge**	**Cost**	**Patients**	**Charge**	**Cost**
Urgent care	30	$170	$5100	70	$170	$11,900
Emergency	70	$750	$52,500	30	$750	$22,500
Referred from UC	27	$750	$20,250	35	$750	$26,250
ED evaluation	67.9	$1000	$67,900	32.5	$1000	$32,500
Inpatient transfer	6.79	$30,000	$203,700	6.79	$30,000	$203,700
TOTAL COST			$349,450			$296,850
Intervention			$0		$250	$25,000
Cost/patient			$3495			$3269
Savings %						7.9%

Table 1.
Economic model.

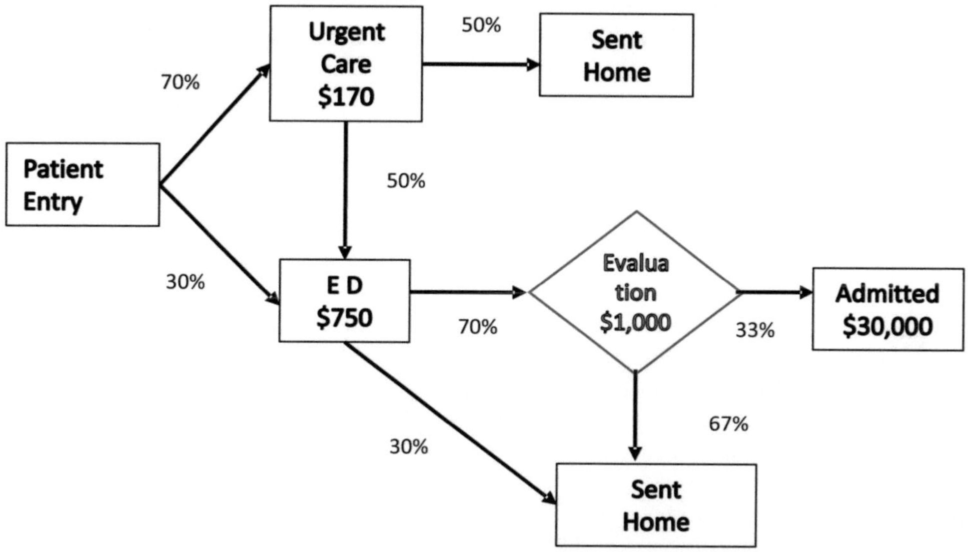

Figure 5.
Proposed patient pathway.

The Economic Model (**Table 1**) illustrates the estimation of the value created by the sample intervention illustrated in the pathways in **Figure 5**, which moves patients from the Emergency Dept. to Urgent Care, as well as more accurately identifies those patients that may safely be sent home after evaluation.

Combining the predicted savings with the cost of delivery of the program allows the Provider/HCM to price its intervention in a manner that allows an appropriate margin for the HCM while also generating an acceptable ROI for the payer. The economic model also allows the HCM to price its contract: in this example the projected savings after intervention charges is 7.9% of projected costs. For a 50/50 gainsharing contract the HCM could each expect savings of 3.95%. This is a point estimate, however, subject to considerable volatility. Before entering into a contract the parties will want to evaluate the uncertainty around the point estimate, which we discuss next.

3.3 Step 3: risk assessment

In Step 2 we created the current and proposed patient pathways, estimated the value created by the HCM and the basic pricing parameters. However, this estimate is a mean; we do not know the variance around the estimated outcome. Variance estimation is important for healthcare models: healthcare claims are highly variable for two reasons. First, the distribution of healthcare claims itself is a convolution of two highly-variable distributions, frequency and severity. Second, outcomes of a healthcare program are subject to performance risk. Step 3 begins with modeling the distribution of the predicted outcome. Additionally, there are multiple variables involved in the predicted outcome; many of these variables can be controlled in order to limit the contract risk. The Risk Assessment step helps the analyst to understand the contribution of individual variables to the predicted outcome and to choose values in such as way as to mitigate some of the inherent stochastic risk of the contracted outcome. **Figure 6** shows some of the variables that comprise a value-based contract that an analyst should consider when modeling contract risk.

Figure 6 shows that designing a value-based contract is a complex undertaking. While we will not discuss all the variables in **Figure 6**, we will discuss some key variables and use them to illustrate the complexity of the modeling that is required as part of the Value-based Contract pricing.

- **Attribution:** it is important to define precisely those patients for which the HCM or provider will accept risk, and at what point the patient is triggered into the risk group. Attribution can occur on a population basis (for example patients with diabetes) or an episode basis (for example knee surgery). Triggers for these patients generally occur within claims datasets. Occasionally triggers may also be found in electronic medical records (although the lack of integrated medical record/claims data makes modeling difficult in this context). Attribution may also be triggered by the use of a derived marker, for example a grouper model (in the US, Hierarchical Condition Categories (HCCs) or Episode Groupers (for example ETGs)). It is also necessary to use triggers to determine which provider should have accountability for a given patient.

Opportunity

Claims sources and suitability
Payer type (MA, Commercial)
Target Condition/Co-morbidities
Condition Definitions (standard or custom)
Condition Inclusions & Exclusions
Claims Inclusions & Exclusions
Eligibility Inclusions & Exclusions
Episode/bundle/pathway logic

Economic Model

Proposed intervention
Intervention Cost
Contract type (bundle/capitation/ Gain-sharing)
Attribution: triggers; timing; exclusions and inclusions (members, claims, eligibility)
Stop Loss/Outliers/Reinsurance
Savings Estimates (PMPM/ROI/MLR improvements)
Attribution: Patient-to provider
Provider to HCM ("affiliation")

Contract Risk Assessment

Measurement Accuracy Modeling
Risk Mitigation: truncation; corridors; duration; study size; inclusions and exclusion rules; reserving analysis; true-up periods; risk adjustment specificity

Contract Terms

Risk/acuity adjustment (standard or custom)
Risk corridors/margin
Quality measures/ outcomes
Surplus/deficit calculation
Gain-share terms: Share/ settlement logic
Calculation performance (internal/external)
HCM and provider payment terms

Outcomes Evaluation

Appropriate and accurate application of contract terms

Figure 6.
Key parameters for a value-based contract.

- **Acuity:** attribution sometimes requires an assessment of patient acuity in cases where the entire population is not managed. Assessment of acuity requires an objective measure such as a predictive model or a grouper model (for example CMS's HCC Model). A provider/HCM should be wary of clients that want to allow physicians or other clinicians referral or patient self-referral into a program because of their lack of objective evaluation and comparability to a control or comparison population.

- **Services:** once the patient population is identified it is important to define precisely those services for which the provider/HCM will accept risk. In all cases the question is whether the provider/HCM accepts risk based on claims for a specific condition only, for a subset of services (e.g. PCP capitation), or for "total cost of care?" In each case there will be valid claims included in the risk pool and exclusions. Exclusions are typically those conditions or services that the provider/HCM does not provide or that are managed by a different provider (for example in the case of a diabetes population, a claim for a cancer diagnosis may be excluded because the HCM will not take risk for a non-diabetes related claim).

- **Baseline and projection:** Many models (the Medicare MSSP ACO model is a good example) rely on comparison of actual outcomes compared with a predicted or projected counter-factual (what would have happened, absent intervention) for the calculation of cost-reduction as the difference between actual and projected costs. A baseline is usually relatively simple to calculate by applying all the contract rules (attribution; services; exclusions etc.) to the payer's data. As a general rule no contracting party should enter into a risk-based contract *without* evaluating the population in actual payer data. Estimating what would have happened to the patient population in the absence of intervention is a challenging task, however. This often requires the projection of a cost "trend" or the expected increase of the cost per patient within the treatment population. There are many sources of trend estimates; the MSSP program uses the experience of a non-treated population, adjusted for differences in average risk as its basis for this calculation.

- **Stop-loss and truncation:** Contracts can be adversely affected by high claim amounts, which occur randomly and unpredictably. For this reason some form of high-cost claim truncation should be considered to limit the contractor's maximum exposure. Truncation results in amounts in excess of the truncation point defaulting to the payer, which may not be acceptable to a payer. As an alternative the provider/HCM could purchase stop-loss insurance making excess amounts above the truncation point (called the "attachment point in a stop-loss contract) the responsibility of the reinsurer. Stop-loss insurance, particularly for many types of value-based contracts tends to be costly because reinsurers lack experience with many of the very specific types of clinical interventions for which reinsurance is sought, which may result in a provider/HCM deciding to accept the risk of high-cost claims itself. If the provider/HCM has adequate financial resources this may not be a bad strategy, but the provider/HCM should not accept the risk without modeling the potential effect of high-cost claims.

- **Risk corridors:** an alternative form of risk mitigation is the risk corridor. We discuss this in more detail, with an example below.

Risk assessment requires simulation of the distribution of outcomes. The provider/HCM will contract at a target rate or price assuming its performance will achieve a particular outcome level. In **Table 1** this was illustrated as $2,969 per patient. The question to be addressed in the Risk Assessment phase is: what is the confidence interval around this estimate and how may variation be mitigated by choosing different values of the parameters in **Figure 6**?

Risk mitigation can be illustrated by looking at an example from the Medicare Shared-savings program, assuming that the provider/HCM is considering a contract with both upside and downside risk. The provider will want to maximize its chance of upside gains and minimize the chance of a downside loss (reimburse Medicare). In a recent studies [10, 17] the authors illustrate that even in the absence of an intervention there is a non-trivial risk that a provider will have to reimburse the payer simply because of the stochastic nature of claims, giving rise to the need for **Risk Corridors**, which are parameters between whose limits no gain or loss is payable.

Figure 7 illustrates this important concept. Note that **Figure 7** illustrates stochastic (claims variability) risk only; in addition, the provider/HCM will be at risk of performance variability as well. **Figure 7** simulates the outcome (calculated savings *assuming no intervention)* of 10,000 samples and shows a relatively wide dispersion around the mean. (The mean is zero in this example because we assume no intervention and therefore no savings effect on the population.) With a corridor, the provider is protected against downside risk at the cost of having to give up the opportunity of a gain on the upside. In the example of **Figure 7**, between 2 and 5% of simulations resulted in losses (reimbursement by the provider/HCM to the payer). The converse is also true: in the majority of cases the imposition of the corridor would have prevented the provider/HCM from receiving a payment despite the HCM having generated savings. If we consider, in addition to the stochastic claims risk, the provider/HCM accepts performance risk as well, the need for sophisticated modeling to understand and mitigate financial risk becomes acute.

One of the biggest challenges for providers/HCMs entering into value-based contracts is population size. This problem has become especially acute in recent years

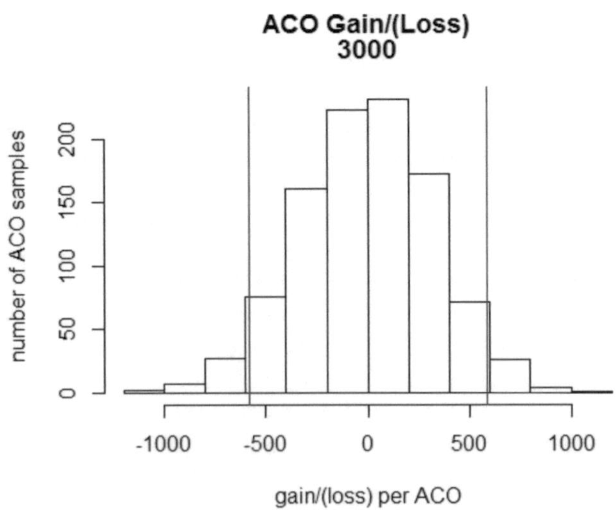

Figure 7.
ACO gain/(loss) distribution: 10,000 simulations.

as providers focus more on specific conditions and sub-populations that may be relatively small or where the condition prevalence results in a small number of target patients. **Figure 7** is an example of a 3,000 life population where a target condition could result in only a few hundred patients being managed. The variance in claims of a few hundred patients is significant; the variance may be mitigated with appropriate truncation and risk corridors but in small samples will remain a major risk to the provider/HCM. A number-needed-to-treat analysis could provide some guidance to the contracting parties regarding their potential variance and risk, but the answer is invariably (except in the case of large insurers) that the provider/HCM will need to manage a much larger population than available to be comfortable with the outcomes. In this case the parties should probably consider an alternative contractual form.

The risk corridor is only one variable that can be modeled; modeling the outcomes using the key variables from **Figure 6** will give the provider/HCM a better idea of the risk that it undertakes and how to mitigate that risk—for example with risk corridors, different attribution definitions, and stop-loss insurance.

3.4 Step 4: contract terms and operationalizing the model

Once the modeling is completed the contract terms will be known and it should be a straightforward matter to prepare a contract. Once the contract is signed, however, it is important that the provider/HMC prepare an implementation and operational plan with appropriate targets, preferably on a monthly basis. Contractors often lose sight of the fact that they are managing a risk contract, often with a one-year term. If the contractor does not adhere to a plan and falls behind, however, it is often impossible to make up patient engagement and cost-reduction numbers later in the contract year. For this reason a projection of the ultimate results and likely reconciliation on a regular basis is important. For some providers/HCMs (particularly those that are publicly traded) an estimate of the final gain/(loss) will also be required because of the need to set up a balance sheet reserve for any ultimate payable or receivable, and to demonstrate revenue recognition.

Operationalizing the contract also may require sophisticated modeling to identify at-risk patients, alert providers to changes in patient status and report on clinical gaps and gap closure. Delivery of programs that rely on clinical resources is also costly and requires that the contractor maximize efficiency. A workflow system incorporating the latest real-time information for providers (if they are managing patients) or patients (self-management) is essential for efficiency and for achieving contracted outcomes. Monitoring the progress of the contract against the plan and reporting on the key performance indicators identified at Step 2 is essential to achieving successful outcomes.

3.5 Step 5: evaluate outcomes

Some models are relatively simple to administer and reconcile: capitated contracts for example may require no reconciliation because the provider is paid a capitated amount from which the provider derives its margin. Shared savings and bundled payment models, on the other hand, can be complicated to reconcile. One challenge with this type of contract is that reconciliation requires complete data, meaning that run-out claims[5] are included in the calculation. Allowing for run-out often imposes

[5] Claims for which services have been rendered but which have either not yet been submitted or, if submitted, have not yet been paid.

a delay of 6 months or more post-contract period before complete claims are available. Reconciliation also requires the application of key contract terms: attribution, services, inclusions/exclusions, truncation and corridors etc.

Because value-based contracts are often very different from contract to contract, payers may need to administer contracts manually. This makes final reconciliation difficult both in terms of actual calculation and payments. Reconciliation payments may be delayed as much as 2 years from contract inception. A provider/HCM will need to plan for this delay in receipt of revenue, and have sufficient capital to carry through to the final reconciliation.

4. Payments

Payments are an important part of the Value-based Contract. They represent the result of an intervention, and being part of the operation of the contract, are not a component of the five analytical steps discussed above. Their importance to a contractor and a payer, however, make it important to discuss payments.

A successful contract will result in a payment from the payer to the provider/HCM. Some models such as capitation and bundled payments result in prospective payments: the provider/HCM receives a fixed amount and there is usually no reconciliation or further exchange of funds. For performance-based contracts such as shared-savings or pay-for-performance, a reconciliation will be necessary to calculate amounts owed or owing. Administration of claims for these contracts can be complicated because providers will submit claims in the normal way to the payer, who must then turn off payment (because the provider will be reimbursed from a pool of funds at reconciliation). It is clearly not satisfactory to the provider/HCM to wait 18 months for reimbursement. The challenge of administering partial payments (or payments after the fact) from a typical claims system, particularly in a payer with multiple different contracts, can be challenging to the payer. In many cases these contracts are administered manually. Solutions such as the application of Stochastic Control processes, in which the ultimate settlement payment is continually estimated and payments are made on account of the ultimate payments offer some promise as a way to satisfy provider/HCM need for near real-time payments. That, however, is a topic for a different chapter.

5. Conclusion

Value-based contracts offer providers of healthcare services an opportunity for higher rewards than traditional payment models, but with considerable additional risk. Risk comes in many forms, from definitions to execution. This chapter has not touched on performance risk, which is the province of other professionals, mostly clinical. But aside from clinical risk a provider/HCM that accepts value-based risk is open to numerous other forms of risk. The good news is that with appropriate planning and modeling these risks can be managed and mitigated. Doing so will allow the provider or healthcare management organization to capitalize on a growing trend in healthcare finance.

DOI: http://dx.doi.org/10.5772/intechopen.103021

Author details

Ian Duncan
Department of Statistics and Applied Probability, University of California Santa Barbara, Santa Barbara, CA, USA

*Address all correspondence to: iduncan@sbactuaries.com

References

[1] Nelson L. In: Congressional Budget Office, editor. Lessons from Medicare's Demonstration Projects on Disease Management and Care Coordination. Washington DC: CBO; 2012

[2] Peikes D, Brown R, Chen A, Schore J. Third Report to Congress on the Evaluation of the Medicare Coordinated Care Demonstration. Princeton, NJ: Mathematica Policy Research; 2008

[3] Peikes D et al. Effects of care coordination on hospitalization, quality of care, and health care expenditures among Medicare beneficiaries: 15 randomized trials. JAMA. 2009;**301**(6):603-618

[4] Berwick D et al. The triple aim: Care, health, and cost. Health Affairs. 2008;**27**(3):759-769

[5] McGlynn EA, Asch S, Adams J, Keesey J, Hicks J, DeCristofaro A, et al. The quality of health care delivered to adults in the United States. New England Journal of Medicine. 2003;**348**:2635-2645

[6] Werner RM, Emanuel E, Pham HH, Navath AS. The future of value-based payment: A Road Map to 2030. In: LDI-HTI Next Decade of Payment Innovation Working Group. Philadelphia, PA: Leonard Davis Institute for Health Economics University of Pennsylvania; 2021

[7] Duncan I. Managing and Measuring Healthcare Intervention Programs. 2nd ed. Winsted, CT: Actex Publications; 2014. p. 446

[8] Marrufo G et al. In: Division of Data Research and Analytic Methods, editor. CMS Bundled Payments for Care Improvement Initiative Models 2-4: Year 7 Evaluation & Monitoring Annual Report. Lewin Group Falls Church VA; 2021. p. 71

[9] United States Congress. Patient Protection and Affordable Care Act, U.S. Congress, Editor. 2010: Washington D.C

[10] Duncan I, Mackenzie AJ, Bonfiglio E, Wrigley T, Liao X. Shared savings model risk in the MSSP Program. North American Actuarial Journal. 2022:1-11 [ePub ahead of Print]. DOI: 10.1080/10920277.2021.1993927

[11] Ternay J. Roadmaps to Value-based Profitability: A Practice Transformation Guide. Centennial Colorado: Medical Group Management Association; 2019. p. 250

[12] Porter ME, Teisberg EO. Re-defining Healthcare: Creating Value-Based Competition on Results. Boston, MA: Harvard Business School Press; 2006

[13] Porter ME. What is value in health care? NEJM. 2010;**363**(26):2477-2481

[14] Terrell GE, Bobbitt JD. Value-Based Healthcare and Payment Models: Including Frontline Strategies for 20 Clinical Subspecialties. Washington DC: American Association of Physician Leadership Inc.; 2020

[15] Dlugacz YD. Value-Based Healthcare: Linking Finance and Quality. San Francisco CA: Jossey-Bass; 2010

[16] Moriates C, Arora V, Shah N. Understanding Value-Based Healthcare. New York NY: McGraw-Hill; 2015

[17] Mackenzie AJ, Teppema S, Wang J, Duncan I. Payment accuracy in value-based care contracts. Austin Medical Sciences. 2021;**6**(3):1-5

Chapter 10

Socio-Economic Considerations of Universal Health Coverage: Focus on the Concept of Health Care Value and Medical Treatment Price

Tomoyuki Takura

Abstract

Healthcare systems generally help improve clinical outcomes by increasing public financial investment. Reasonable policymaking is crucial for identifying the financial burden involved, and analytical tools related to the relationship between universal health coverage (UHC) and socio-economic factors are essential. This study, along with the context and reports related to health insurance systems, examines the financial mechanisms that support UHC and the economic factors that dominate the clinical outcomes that benefit from it. The first section examines the socio-economic factors that affect universal coverage. Examples of methods for quantitatively evaluating the relationships and their analysis results are also summarized. The subsequent section summarizes the concept of medical value and the methodology for its evaluation, which are indispensable for examining the appropriate development of medical insurance systems. Research cases related to the significance of lifesaving and drug discovery are introduced, considering the possibility of allocating public resources. In the final section, the concept of price formation, which also considers medical value, is organized from the perspective of economics and medicine, with the optimization of medical treatment behavior in mind. For example, a report that analyzes the factors of price levels, focusing on Japanese private practices, is introduced.

Keywords: medical fee, value of medicine, health insurance, cost accounting, cost-effectiveness, service coverage index, gross domestic product, health expenditure, poverty, population, utility theory, nephrotic syndrome, childbirth

1. Introduction

Answers regarding the value of a medical system can vary depending on various considerations and degrees of interest. Even when considering the universal values of human life and health, their implications are presumed to depend both on the sense of individual values and a country's history, culture, national character, and surrounding socioeconomics [1, 2]. Meanwhile, if we discuss human dignity's ethical and moral aspects, the fundamental values of health and life typically exhibit a consensus within the minimum necessary basic range. In other words, the value of the medical system can be considered a mechanism for stable supply (cultivation of a sense of security) that guarantees basic human rights. Given the socio-economic background, the significance of discussing the medical insurance systems of countries from this perspective has recently been increasing. Under these circumstances, the World Health Organization (WHO) has promoted universal health coverage (UHC).

UHC refers to universal access to all people for necessary healthcare services—irrespective of time, place, and their financial condition. UHC, a goal that the healthcare system must strive to achieve, includes basic health services: promotion, prevention, treatment, rehabilitation, and palliative care. This goal takes the civic perspective. Given this background, the understanding and contribution of all members of society (citizens) is essential to the realization of UHC. Its promotion requires a balance between the benefits and burdens at the citizen level. The aforementioned value trends were involved in discussing this balance. In other words, the choices and decisions of individuals and groups are influenced by values. However, issues related to equity and efficiency exist in allocating resources for public goods. The significance of applying value theory and market principles, although limited, has been discussed for a long time [3].

Therefore, the political dimension is also important when considering UHC progress. To promote UHC, some issues regarding evaluating the medical insurance system must be resolved. The increasing importance of socio-economic measures in medical insurance systems has attracted considerable attention. In general, the following three issues have been addressed: (1) The perspective through which the medical insurance system's outcomes (goals and significance) must be discussed and evaluated. (2) The measurement and analysis of the impact of socio-economic factors on health insurance system outcomes. (3) Determining the operation of the medical insurance system (e.g., benefits and burdens, allocation of resources) based on the aforementioned issues. Each issue has a broad and complex context; thus, consistent effort is required.

The development of public medical resources, especially the financial investment system (national burden and insured burden), is indispensable for the sustainable operation of the medical system. Therefore, an analysis of the characteristics of each country's political systems is required. As rational policy decision-making is imperative for discussing the financial burden, analytical tools such as those presented in this chapter are necessary. For example, in future studies, a cost-effectiveness analysis (CEA) could be conducted. Additionally, adopting a longitudinal research design (panel data analysis) would make it possible to account for the effects of fluctuations in external factors—such as the real economy—with high accuracy. For example, a report suggests that it is important to optimize resource allocation from the perspective of public interest rather than simply increasing the medical expenses per capita to develop the medical insurance system [4].

Based on the above, harmonizing the public and private sectors is a theme in healthcare insurance systems. This coincides with harmonizing the benefits and burdens of healthcare policy between individuals and society. This requires a macroeconomic analysis of the relationship between health sector outcomes and socio-economic factors. Therefore, this approach also involves financial aspect and discusses the relationship between the real economy and public interest activities. Regarding healthcare services, there is a lot of discussion about payment formulas and price levels in the relationship between stakeholders (economic payers, providers, and service recipients) [5–16]. In other words, there are themes related to the proper allocation of social security funds and the improvement of inefficiencies in the public market. Therefore, a microanalysis is essential in the discussion of healthcare insurance systems. From this perspective, utility theory and welfare economics are applied to elucidate the mechanisms of price formation and treatment selection behavior.

In particular, these themes are becoming more important in the quasi-public medical market, such as Japan's universal health insurance system, medical resources consisting of social premiums, general taxes (including subsidies), and patient out-of-pocket expenses. For example, rising drug prices and procedure fees have a structure that rebounds from social and individual burdens. Therefore, the significance of comprehensively discussing phenomena and issues that straddle both macro- and micro-aspects has been emphasized (**Figure 1**). For example, high expectations for cost-effectiveness evidence can be applied to macro- and micro-issues to ensure the sustainability of the system and the appropriateness of resource allocation. From the above, three closely-related perspectives will be discussed: an examination of UHC considering socio-economic factors, examination of the significance of citizens' value in resource allocation, and examination of price formation considering patients' economic burden.

This chapter explains the concept of the approach required to address the aforementioned issues and introduces examples of related research reports as a guidepost for discussions in the areas concerned. In the first section, the socio-economic factors that affect UHC are examined, and examples of quantitatively evaluating these relationships and their analysis results are provided. Subsequently, the concepts of medical value and methodology, which are indispensable to the ideal development of the medical insurance system, are summarized. Research cases related to the significance of lifesaving and drug discovery are introduced, considering the possibility of allocating public resources. In the final section, the concept of price (fee, charge) formation, which also considers medical value, is organized based on the characteristics of economics and medicine. For example, a report that analyzes the mechanism of price levels, focusing on Japanese private practice (out-of-pocket), is introduced.

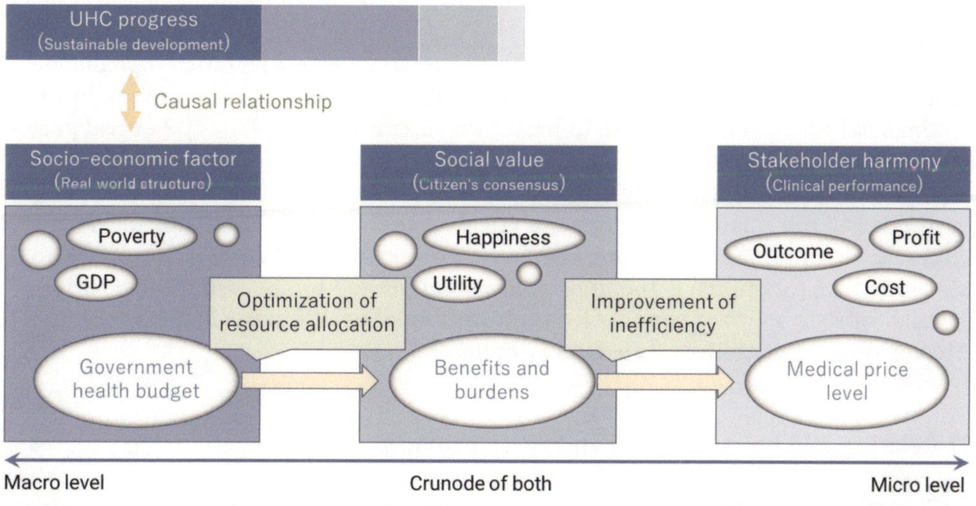

Figure 1.
Three closely related perspectives are examined: An examination of UHC considering socio-economic factors, the significance of citizens' value in resource allocation, and price formation considering the economic burden of patients. Note: UHC, universal health coverage.

2. Progress in UHC: socio-economic impact

2.1 Concept of UHC and surrounding economic trends

Sustainable Development Goal (SDG) 3 comprises 13 targets related to "health and welfare for all." The other 16 goals were either related—or indirectly contributed—to health. The SDGs aim to "leave no one behind" and are international objectives applicable to developing and advanced countries. UHC is a concept that includes 1) protection from financial risks for all, 2) access to quality primary health services, and 3) access to essential medicines and effective, high-quality, and inexpensive vaccines. Target 3.8 SDG 3, which involves achieving UHC and health improvement worldwide, is considered the most crucial task of the WHO [17].

The measurement approaches and definitions of the UHC index evolved between 2015 and 2019, and the index is now used in every global monitoring report [18]. UHC progress between regions and countries can be compared. Additionally, the UHC service coverage index (SCI) has been calculated as a single number (i.e., score) since the late 2010s, thereby improving comparability between nations. Although the performance of different countries can now be compared, global monitoring alone is insufficient to guide policymaking [19]. Therefore, each country should be encouraged to develop a country-specific global framework. The relationship between the environmental factors surrounding medical care and progress toward UHC should be analyzed to achieve this.

Healthcare systems generally help improve clinical outcomes by increasing public financial investment [20, 21]. Meanwhile, declining birth rates, aging populations, and the maturation of medical systems generally tend to reduce the baseline performance of medical systems. Some reports mention that unemployment and poverty, which are distant causes of catastrophic health costs, are factors that reduce service coverage index levels [22]. Therefore, there is room for countermeasures, including population policies and economic measures. For example, future economic growth strategies could include the promotion of healthcare and life sciences industries. Improvements in health care programs include disease prevention and medical insurance policies.

Problems regarding medical financial systems constitute a significant challenge to achieving UHC. According to the WHO, a healthcare financial system that eliminates the financial constraints of access to health services is crucial [23, 24]. Several previous studies have suggested that UHC is more likely to be achieved when patients' out-of-pocket medical costs are low [25]. As rational policy decision-making is imperative for discussing the financial burden, analytical aspects, such as UHC and socio-economic factor relationships, are necessary. For example, CEA, a performance analysis of medical functions, is the most common approach for assessing the health benefits for each spent or the cost for each additional health unit. CEA is a tool used to enhance the sustainability of medical systems.

2.2 Relationship between UHC and socio-economic factors

This section introduces an example of the relationship between SCI and major socio-economic indicators to establish UHC levels and economic factors [25]. This study used SCI as a proxy for progress toward UHC in 11 Asian countries. A fixed-effects regression model was employed to analyze panel data from 2015 to 2017, and to explain the interrelationship between the SCI and major socio-economic indicators (health expenditure, unemployment, etc.) Performance analysis (to determine the ratio of the achieved SCI level to gross domestic product or health expenditure displacement) was also conducted. This analysis examines the balance between the degree of achievement related to UHC and a country's economic level.

The gross domestic product (GDP) and SCI had a significant positive correlation (Spearman's rank correlation coefficient [Rs] = 0.716, $p < 0.01$). Health expenditure and SCI were significantly and positively correlated (Rs = 0.743, $p < 0.01$). When both GDP and SCI indicators were transformed using logarithms, the abovementioned trend did not change significantly (Rs = 0.731, $p < 0.01$; **Figure 2**). The results of the panel data analysis showed that GDP per capita significantly contributed to SCI (standardized partial regression coefficient, 1.6129; partial regression coefficient, 0.0049; 95% Confidence interval [CI], 0.0025–0.0074; **Table 1**). The total population, governmental health expenditure, unemployment, and poverty rates were statistically significant, whereas health expenditure was not significant. The unemployment and poverty rates show a negative trend, and the entire model is statistically significant ($R^2 = 0.991$, F-test: $p < 0.001$). The ROC curve for health expenditure per GDP for SCI showed a cutoff of 3.7% ($p < 0.01$) for the Youden index and 4.9% ($p < 0.01$) for the shortest distance (AUC = 0.8125, 95% CI: 0.6350–0.9899, $p < 0.05$; **Figure 3**).

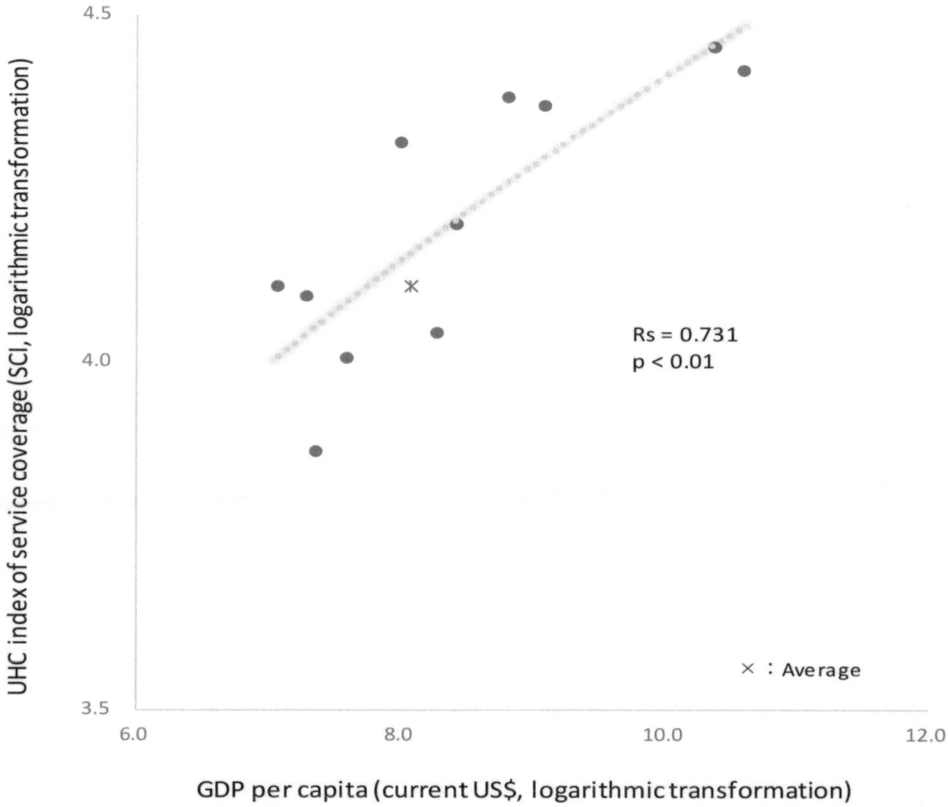

Figure 2.
Relationship between economic level (GDP) and SCI (logarithmic transformation, 2017). Note: UHC, universal health coverage; SCI, service coverage index [21].

UHC index of service coverage (SCI)	Partial regression coefficient	Standardized partial regression coefficient	SE	p-value	95% CI
Population (total: million people)	0.0049	0.1921	0.0012	0.0001	0.0025–0.0074
GDP per capita (current USD)	0.0017	1.6129	0.0002	< 0.001	0.0013–0.0021
Health expenditure (% of GDP)	2.3481	0.4116	1.5748	0.136	−0.7386–5.4347
Government health expenditures (% of general government expenditures)	1.4511	0.6575	0.2804	< 0.001	0.9015–2.0006
Unemployment rate (%: ratio of unemployed persons)	−1.4764	−0.2253	0.7105	0.0377	−2.8689–0.0838
Poverty rate (%: poverty gap)	−1.6736	−0.2303	0.4674	0.0003	−2.5897–0.7575
Model: R^2 = 0.991, F test: $p < 0.001$					

Note: GDP, gross domestic product; UHC, universal health coverage; SCI, service coverage index; SE, standard error; CI, confidence interval [21].

Table 1.
Panel data analysis of the impact of economic level (GDP, health expenditure, unemployment, and poverty) on SCI.

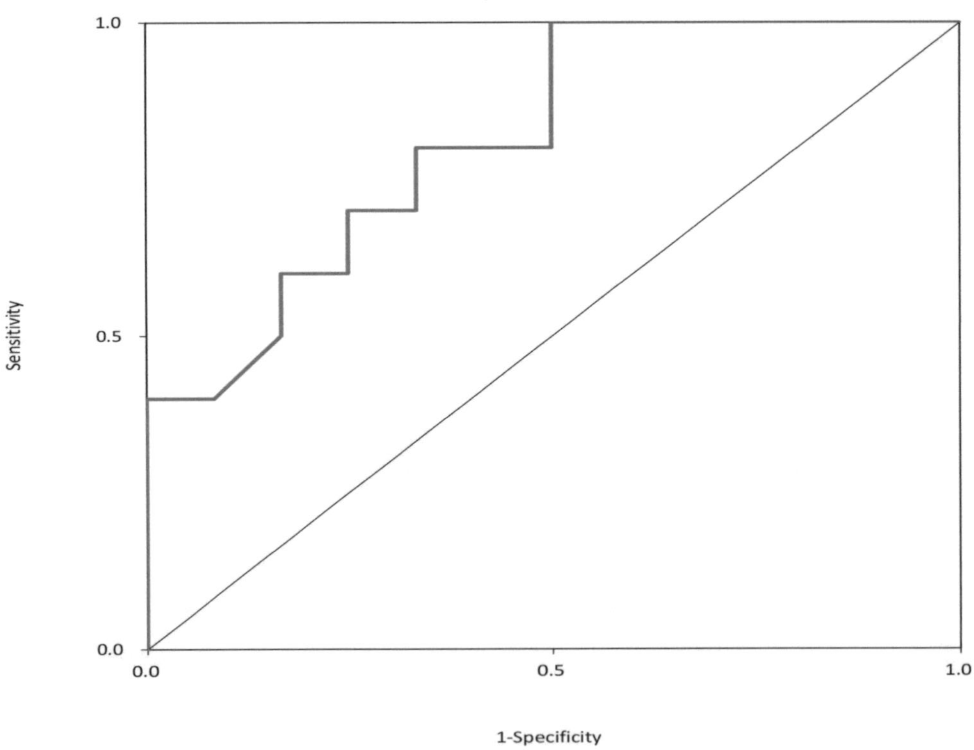

Figure 3.
ROC curve of health expenditure (per GDP: %) for SCI (criterion: Score 70) [21].

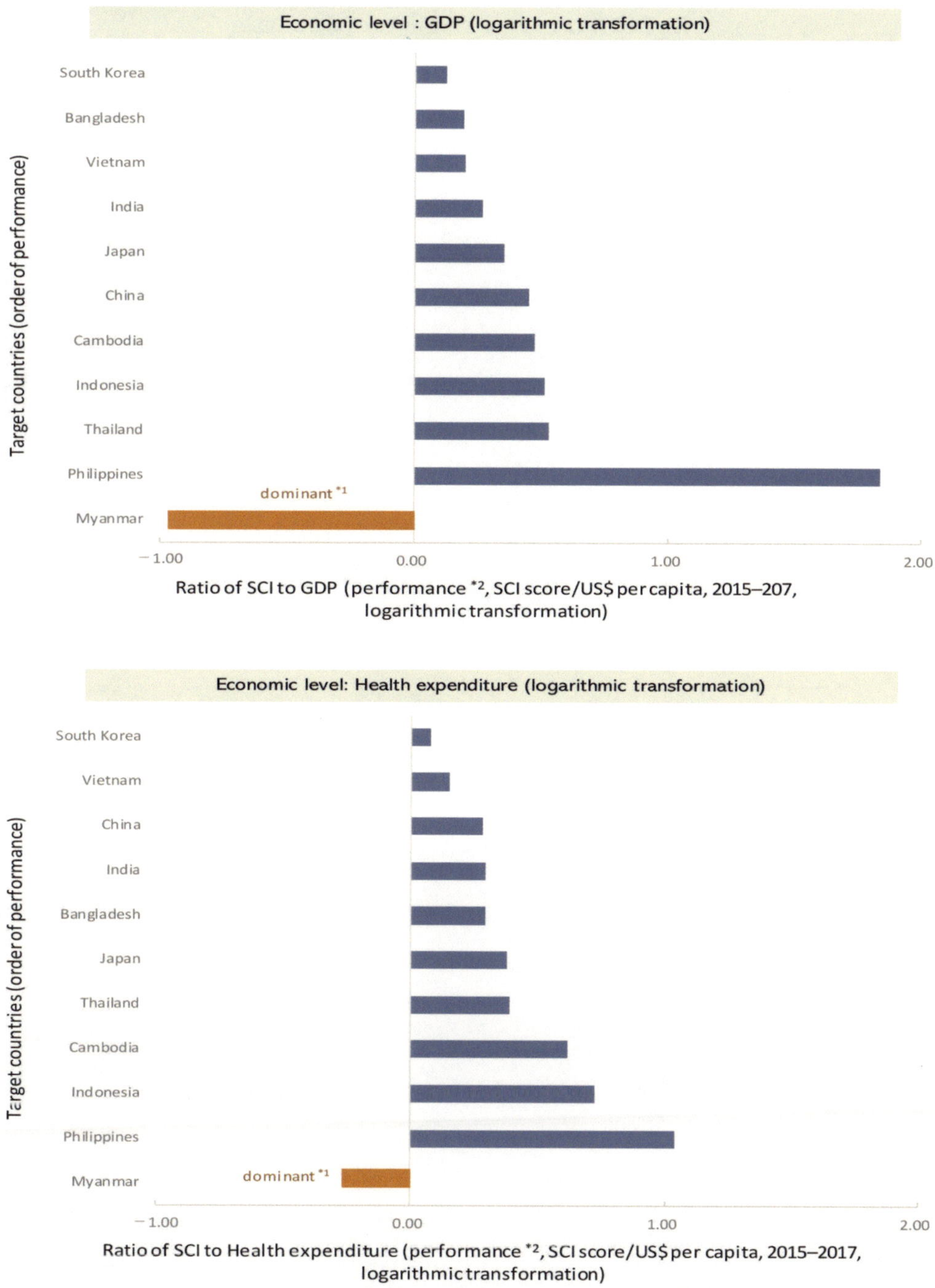

Figure 4.
*Performance status by country (broad cost-effectiveness analysis based on displacement from 2015 to 2017). Note: SCI, service coverage index. *1: Dominant is positioned in a more cost-effective dimension with increasing outcomes (SCI) even if the economy (GDP) declines. *2: Performance was a cost-effectiveness analysis (difference in outcome "SCI" ÷ difference in the economy "GDP"; displacement from 2015 to 2017). Both indices were logarithmically transformed to consider the elasticity [21].*

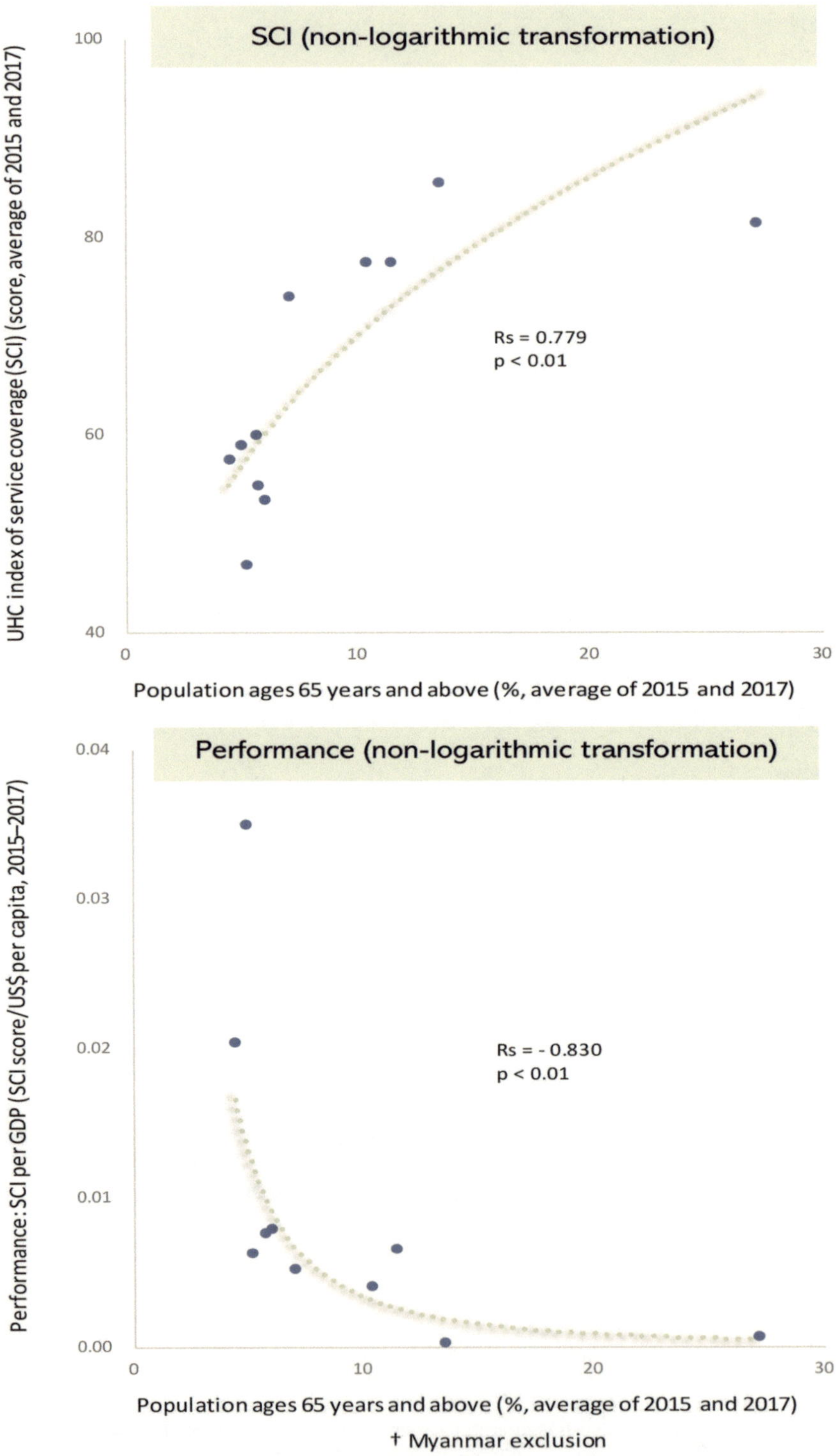

Figure 5.
Trends in SCI and performance (economic level: GDP) with respect to the aging rate (percentage of the population aged 65 years and above). Note: UHC, universal health coverage; SCI, service coverage index. (†) Myanmar has a different quadrant (dimension) because it is "dominant" [21].

From the results of the performance analysis after the logarithmic transformation of each index, South Korea (high-income country: HIC) scored the lowest (GDP: 0.12 SCI score/USD per capita, health expenditure: 0.07 SCI score/USD per capita; **Figure 4**), followed by Vietnam (lower-middle-income country: LMIC) and India (LMIC). Japan's (HIC) performance was moderate, while Indonesia (UMIC), Thailand (UMIC), and Cambodia (LMIC) had relatively high performance. The Philippines (LMIC) had the highest performance (GDP: 1.84 SCI score/USD per capita, health expenditure: 1.04 SCI score/USD per capita). Myanmar (LMIC) was marked as the "dominant quadrant." The more effective but less expensive quadrant exhibited the best performance in the cost-effectiveness analysis. When the relationship between the proportion of the population aged 65 and above was organized without logarithmic conversion, the SCI score increased with age ($Rs = 0.779$, $p < 0.01$), and the performance value decreased ($Rs = -0.830$, $p < 0.01$; **Figure 5**).

Each of the four SCI components had a different level of achievement (**Figure 6**). LMICs were most countries with SCI levels of 60 or below (i.e., Bangladesh, India, Indonesia, and Cambodia), where "infectious diseases" and "service capacity and access" were more widely dispersed. This was compared to the group of countries with SCIs of more than 80 (i.e., South Korea, Japan, Thailand, and China), HIC, and UMIC. Multiple regression analysis used SCI's annual rate of change as the objective variable and SCI components as the explanatory variable. The results indicate that "service capacity and access" significantly contributed to the SCI level (standardized partial regression coefficient, 0.9209; partial regression coefficient, 0.3581; 95% CI, 0.3142–0.4019). Furthermore, when the GDP per capita and "service capacity and access" values of each country were relatively arranged, with Japan as the standard, a positive correlation was observed between the two indicators (i.e., single correlation: $Rs = 0.901$, $p < 0.01$) (**Figure A1**).

2.3 Health economies necessary for the development of UHC

The present study used SCI as a proxy for the progress of UHC. Currently available service coverage metrics focused on infectious diseases and reproductive, neonatal, maternal, and child health [26]. In this study, the indicators for SCI-related data (**Figure A2**) were "reproductive, maternal, newborn and child health," "infectious diseases," "noncommunicable diseases," and "service capacity and access." In addition, the country-by-country socio-economic indicators included "total population," "population aged 65 and above," "gross domestic product (GDP) per capita," "health expenditure per GDP/per capita," "government health expenditures," "unemployment rate," and "poverty rate." All data were converted into a panel from 2015 to 2017; SCI-related and socio-economic data were also compiled [27–29].

According to the analysis results derived by applying these data, UHC progress tends to increase as the share of the healthcare domain in government spending increases. Future studies on UHC development measures are important to discuss the appropriate form of resource allocation (public finance) according to sustainability-based productivity and efficiency or value evaluation (national consensus). Based on the statistical analysis results, some cases exist wherein SCI achievement levels differ even among countries at the same economic level. Furthermore, SCI improvement is small, even in countries with high economic investment levels. Exploring these factors and considering improvement measures are assumed to promote UHC progress. This study examined the influences of the maturity of the medical system as an additional country-specific factor (rather than the social system, national character, and culture).

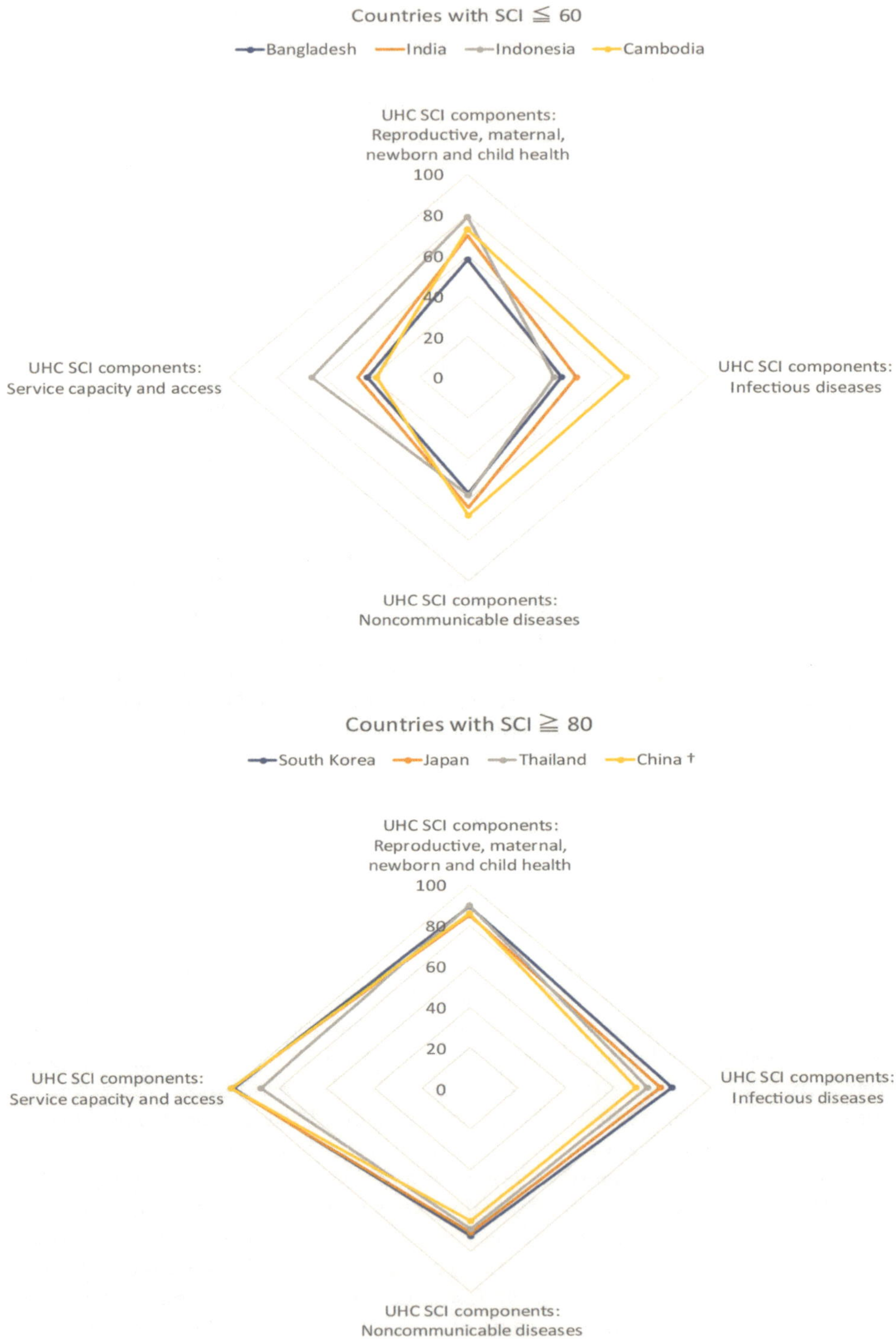

(†) China has an SCI of 79, but it is shown because it is as close as possible to the relevant group.

Figure 6.
Distribution composition of SCI components according to SCI level (≥ 60 and ≥ 80). Note: SCI, service coverage index [21].

The results showed that when aging and health expenditure exceed a certain level, UHC performance decreases as a country's need to raise its goal increases. Additionally, the weight of "service capacity and access" to SCI was considerable. This secondary index, which embodies the environment of the healthcare system, can be considered a surrogate index that predicts the maturity of social and medical care. The considerable impact of these factors on UHC implies that stable development cannot be expected simply by expanding the expenditure scale due to the mechanisms related to economic conditions. As a result, policymakers must implement countermeasures based on indicators that can estimate the economic status of the UHC approach, such as its cost-effectiveness.

CEA is often applied to medical-economic evaluations, such as high-priced medicines and health programs, but can also be applied to macro issues, such as medical systems [30]. Cost-effectiveness is an instrument widely used in Western health systems. The instrument provides the information needed to reach a consensus among stakeholders in allocating medical resources and setting medical prices. As UHC progress requires country-specific efforts, as discussed in the introduction, estimating the coefficients that define each country's UHC progress and socio-economic status is also necessary. Hence, a country-specific performance analysis (CEA: country-specific coefficient calculations) was conducted. In the present study, CEA was performed using economic level as a cost index and SCI level as an effective index.

This approach suggests that regardless of the maturity of the system or the size of the economy, the status of UHC activities in each country can be evaluated based on the displacement of economic and SCI levels achieved.

3. Concept and calculation method of medical value: cost-utility application

3.1 Background related to medical value

This section summarizes the conditions and mechanisms of the link between value and price discussion in a medical system.

In a private economy, where the market principle works, goods (and services) are demanded and supplied in the market based on people's decision-making (free choice and action) depending on changes in price levels. If the market works well, supply and demand will be balanced, and various goods will be properly distributed. The relationship between benefits and burdens in this market is easy to explain. Meanwhile, in a public economy, where the government is the main operator, the market principle works in a limited way. Taxes that enforce the burden are a receiver of supply costs for the demand of goods.

Therefore, public needs and expenditures (including reallocation) are generally determined by the government's judgment. However, price levels in the public economy are often formed by costs (e.g., size of spending budget), which are both inefficient and inconsistent with market utility (i.e., consumer satisfaction). Additionally, the allocation of public resources may deviate from the balance between supply and demand, and inequity among participants within a group may be promoted. Thus, issues related to Use-value, Marginal utility, and Pareto optimization become apparent in the public economy [31, 32].

Subsequently, the concept of verifying the economic appropriateness of the market function and product price (among others) arises by balancing the number of resources consumed and the results obtained (e.g., cost-effectiveness and performance) [2]. As an example of its widespread use, considering large-scale public investments (e.g., the construction of dams and bridges), the desirability of the project's implementation is evaluated based on its cost-effectiveness. Additionally, in the private economy, where technological innovation is active, and consumers have numerous choices, the concept of cost-effectiveness is used more actively to incorporate activities and stimulate product appeal. Consequently, the basic and broad concept of cost-effectiveness has developed in social policy decision-making and resource management fields. Its know-how has been cultivated in contract society and management activities and used in social consensus-building and decision-making.

Meanwhile, the provision of medical services is characterized by information asymmetry and restrictions on opportunity costs (options) against the background of health and life. Therefore, healthcare markets differ from common markets that exhibit typical demand and supply; this market has three parties (citizens, insurance, and providers) and faces asymmetric information that creates several market problems (i.e., common equilibrium market laws do not apply), including problems in defining prices. Although this is inherently unfair (bias) in the health sector from the perspective of citizens' financial burden, the system is based on medical needs such that the needs of the patient, regardless of the outcomes, receive the same medical care. Since such a tendency threatens the system's sustainability, there have been attempts to improve it as much as possible by utilizing cost-effectiveness and utility theory.

By their very nature, public goods are non-competitive; therefore, the role of price tends to be smaller. Medical care has restrictions on individual choice. However, CEA (including cost-utility analysis [CUA]) is widely used to evaluate medical technology in high-income countries, and prices are determined according to this evaluation. Recently, pricing has become more common with evidence-based or value-based approaches. In this method, a consumer's natural internal decision-making regarding consumption behavior is externally substituted by other stakeholders under certain conditions (typically advocating the maximization of group benefits) for a certain group or system based on the law of equal marginal utility and expected utility theory. These methods will be considered along with the uncertainty of outcomes and limited rationality of human beings.

The medical systems of many countries have historically operated as part of the social security system, as they gather high public interest from the necessity for all people. Further, against the background of stable supply, the pricing of medical services has often been based on costs. As described in the previous section, numerous developed countries face structural issues, such as declining birth rates, aging populations, and rising costs of medical services; thus, verification of price levels has become an urgent concern [25]. Therefore, the need to build a social consensus on the economic burden of the value of medical services has been increasing, and the verification of price levels while considering cost-effectiveness has further expanded [33]. Against this background, discussions on value evaluation and price levels in the medical field are being conducted using various approaches to consider cost-effectiveness.

3.2 Calculation method of medical value

Utility refers to the degree of subjective satisfaction or demand fulfillment that each consumer obtains when consuming a certain good or service and is considered a fundamental concept in economics [34]. When interpreted broadly, human economic activities and all human behaviors (including the selection of medical services) aim to maximize the utility to be acquired as the background. Thus, this concept can explain the background of stakeholder behavior changes (e.g., decisions and choices) in the field of health care [35]. Furthermore, a method supported by varied theories related to utility was assumed as an approach to value evaluation.

In summary, "value" is regarded as the meaning of the existence (usefulness or significance in a narrow sense) of an object regardless of whether it is "tangible or intangible." For example, in the public sector, meaning is often organized using exchange value and use-value. A value is diverse and difficult to quantify in general; however, it should be explained to the parties concerned (**Figure 7**) [36] when discussing it as part of a social system. This perspective is even more important for the effective utilization (fair distribution) of public properties. Aspects related to life and health should first be discussed from the perspective of "use-value" in developing society. Furthermore, medical care is expected to be provided to everyone at a fairly low cost (public aspect).

Therefore, several countries worldwide have more or less developed the medical field as a public system, following the lead of the 1978 Alma Ata Declaration. Specifically, Japan's universal health insurance system is assumed to have experienced this trend (see **Figure 8**). However, highly specialized professionals and therapeutic materials require large investments in developing medical resources, and their supply is restricted. Therefore, to operate and develop medical care as a social system—considering the "exchange value" content that accompanies scarcity and building a

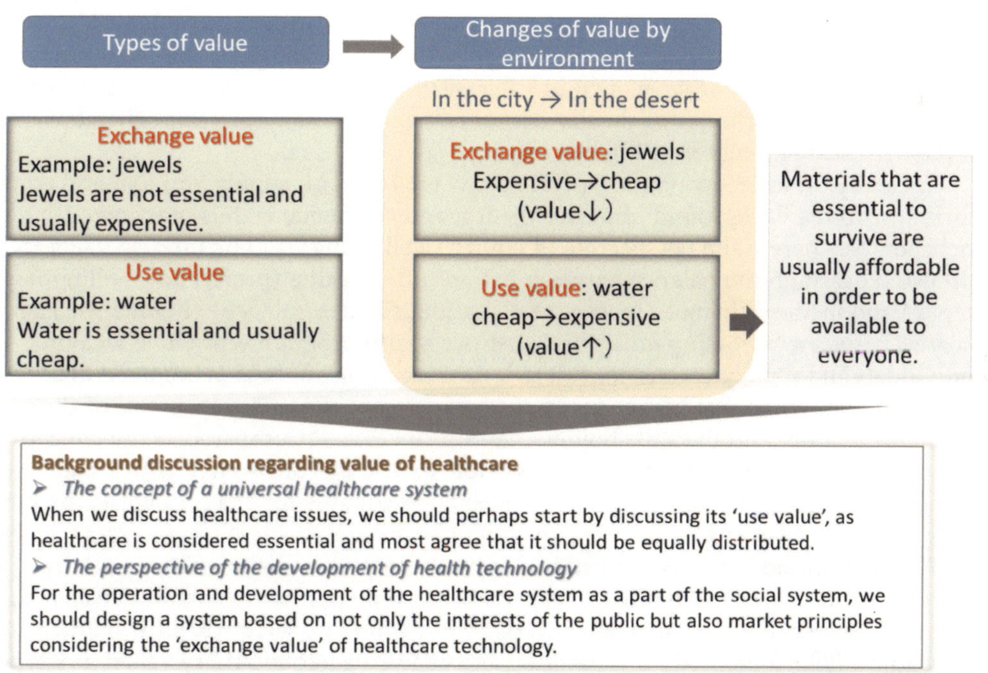

Figure 7.
The conception of value assessment in the quasi-public healthcare system: The balance of the valuation of technical innovations and the guarantee that all patients have access. The public medical marketplace requires a system that considers both use and exchange values [2].

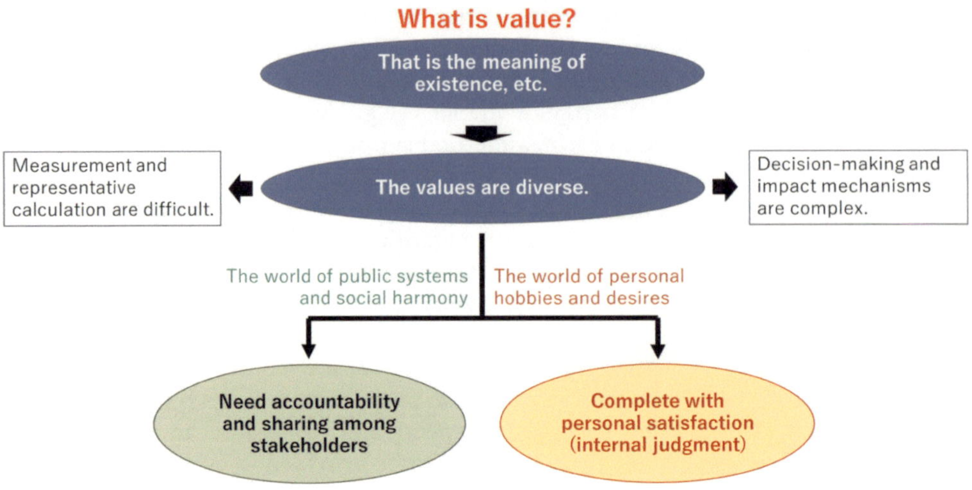

Figure 8.
Significance and key characteristics of value measurement in the public economy (decision-making and resource allocation) [36].

system that incorporates certain market principles (economic aspect)—are crucial [2]. This perspective is also important in discussing consistency within the real economy.

Thus, in a quasi-public healthcare market such as Japan, it is desirable to provide mature and widespread medical care at low-cost while guaranteeing a high economic level for innovative (or effective) medical care and specialized resources. Moreover, a system that balances the use and exchange of values is necessary. As previously mentioned, assessing value in the medical field involves various restrictions. Value evaluation can be performed in several ways, which are inadequate for consistency with the real economy or developed as a theory of price setting. The approach to value evaluation that contributes to the discussion of economic activities and official prices in the healthcare system is as follows:

Generally, in microeconomics, prices converge based on supply and demand equilibrium with the background of utility theory, and efficiency is thus maximized. Incorporating herein the perspective of equity (well-being), public interest value is discussed based on the balance between patient utility value (preference, willingness to pay) and medical finance (income reallocation, finance balance) (**Figure 9**). The balance between increasing utility and cost per health program unit while weaving individuals and society is thus considered. As a result, if utility is maximized in a certain budget range, the higher performance increases the utility in a total of the entire population, and the stakeholders' "value" increases. Compared to the conceptual discussion of value, it is relatively possible to discuss consistency with a real economy or a general value; hence, it is considered suitable for examining the medical price of the public sector.

The value of medical services can be indirectly evaluated in the public sector by applying the marginal utility theory and scales based on preferences while considering different conditions and objectives from those in the private sector [37]. Incidentally, in the medical field, a method for measuring and analyzing patient utility values as a type of health-related quality of life has been developed. The application of this concept to CEA is CUA, which is a type of CEA. Based on the above, the medical value is calculated as "health recovery (patient outcomes such as utility)/resource consumption (direct medical cost) ⇒ medical performance = medical, economic value" [38] (**Figure 10**).

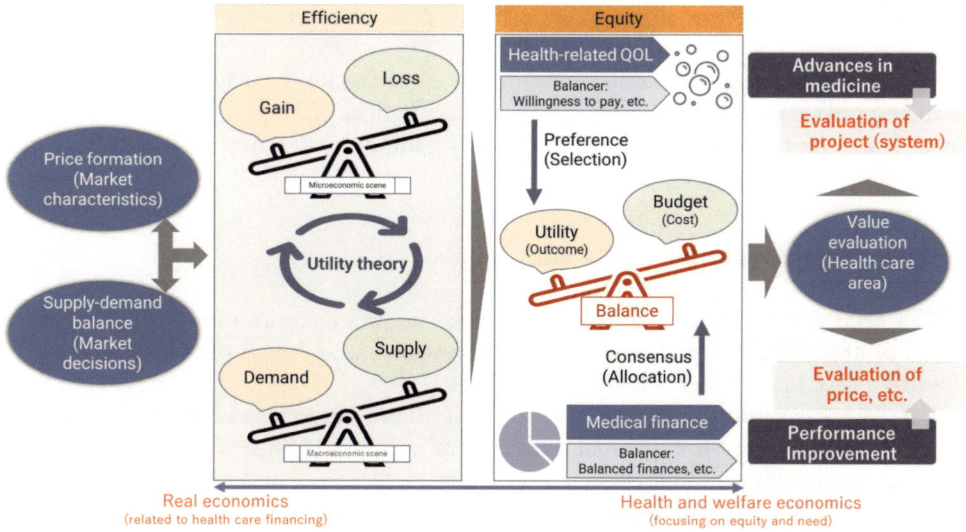

Figure 9.
Concept of value evaluation of health care based on utility theory and cost-effectiveness considering welfare economics.

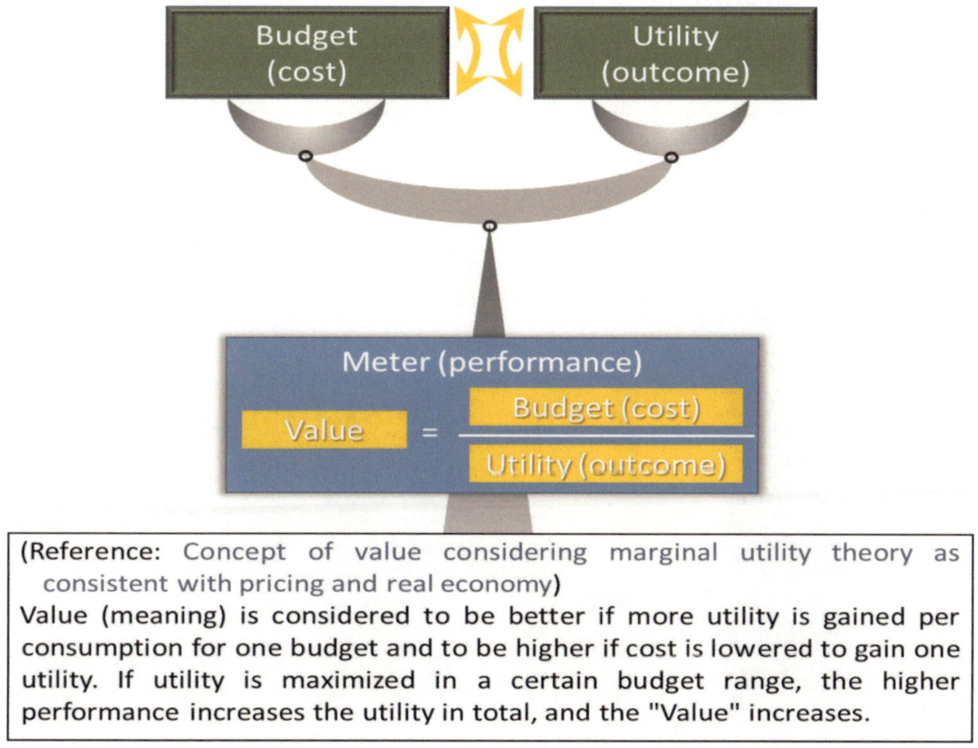

Figure 10.
Concept of economic performance: One of the methods used to discuss the economic value of healthcare. "Value" in social activities is determined by the balance between capital investment and its returns. If a certain amount of money is paid to use a certain service (function), its value is determined by performance, equal to the amount of service (function) divided by the cost. For the consumption of one budget item, the greater the result, the higher is the value. The amount in terms of "restoration of health" is used as an index of "function" in the medical field [2].

A related concrete methodology is cost-effectiveness analysis, which considers health programs' medical and economic position.

This explains the socio-economic significance of the medical services provided by balancing public costs and earned utility in the medical market. It is believed that the higher the performance, the greater the utility (clinical outcomes for patients) as part of the value of the budget range.

3.3 Evaluation cases of medical value

This section introduces reports that discuss the socio-economic significance of the spread of lifesaving medical devices and the research and development (R&D) of expensive pharmaceuticals (at the time of 2010).

First, a case of microeconomic valorization of end-stage renal failure is discussed [39]. With the progression of renal impairment in patients with chronic kidney disease, the dysregulation of electrolyte and water metabolism and retention of uremic toxins can significantly impact health status and even threaten life [40]. Treatment with hemodialysis (HD) should target maintaining the amount and composition of body fluids within the normal range. The study subjects were aged >20 years and had received HD for at least 6 months. HD patients were prospectively observed for 36 months, and patient utility was assessed based on the EQ-5D, from which quality-adjusted life years (QALYs) were estimated. Medical costs were calculated based on the medical service fees. Cost-effectiveness, defined as the incremental cost-utility

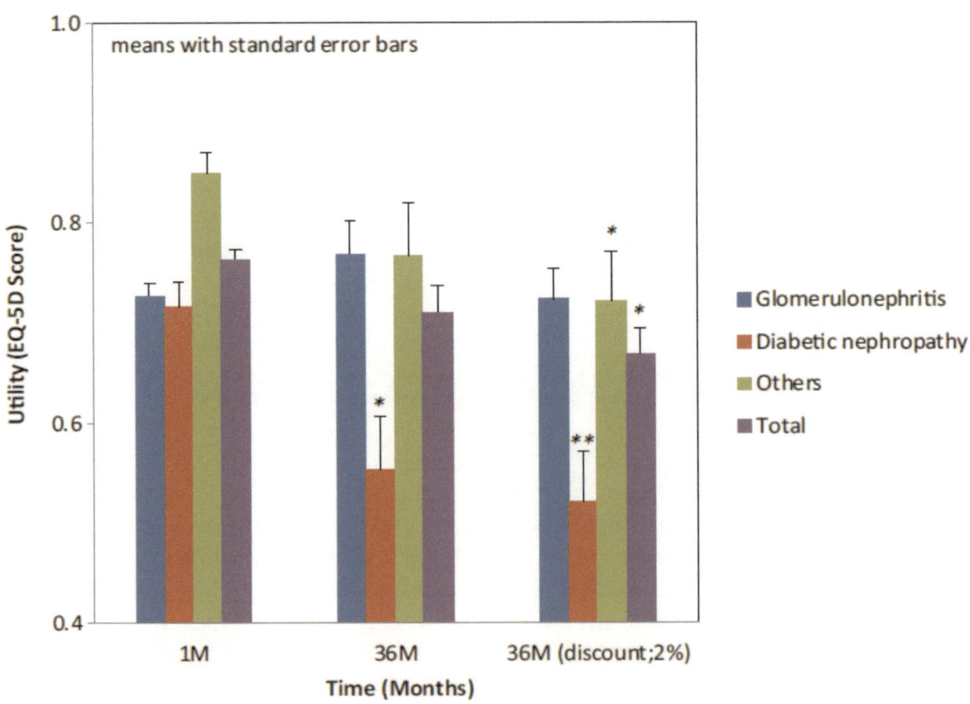

Figure 11.
Utility values (EQ-5D score) during the first 4 weeks of observation and the 36th week. Four-week interval after the classification of primary diseases for end-stage kidney disease (glomerulonephritis, diabetes mellitus, and the whole) [39]. $^{*}p < 0.05$, $^{**}p < 0.01$.

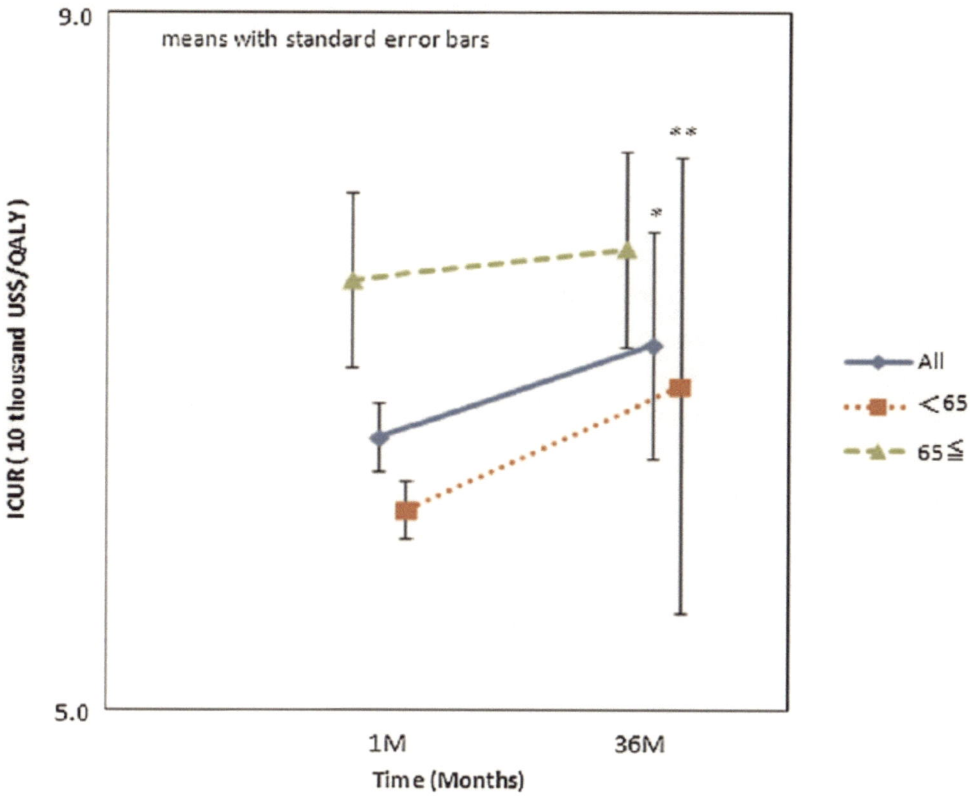

Figure 12.
*Change in cost-effectiveness (ICUR) between the first 4 weeks of observation and the 36th four-week interval. *p < 0.05, **p < 0.01 [39].*

ratio (ICUR), was analyzed socially. A total of 29 patients (mean age; 59.9 ± 13.1 years) undergoing 437 dialysis sessions were analyzed.

Utility-based EQ-5D score was 0.75 ± 0.21, and the estimated total medical cost for 1 year of maintenance HD (MHD) treatment was 45,200 ± 8800 USD. On average, the ICUR was 68,800 ± 44,700 USD/QALY (**Figure 11**). When comparing the ICUR based on the causes of kidney failure, the value for diabetic nephropathy was higher than that for glomerulonephritis (81,700 ± 62,800 vs. 68,200 ± 40,700). The ICUR after 36 months of observation increased mainly in patients below 65 years of age (all $P < 0.05$; <65, $P < 0.01$; ≥ 65, not significant) (**Figure 12**). MHD could improve the socio-economic status of older-adult patients with end-stage kidney disease; however, the ICUR for diabetic nephropathy was higher than that for glomerulonephritis (**Table 2**). However, the ICUR does not deteriorate in older-adult patients. Therefore, measures to prevent malnutrition and establish the optimum time per session and frequency of dialysis (i.e., optimal dialysis volume) are necessary to further improve MHD's cost-effectiveness.

The present findings may contribute to the reexamination of the socio-economic value of MHD therapy, which is a lifesaving medical treatment.

Subsequently, a case of socio-economic valuation of a (then) new drug for the refractory nephrotic syndrome was discussed [41]. Nephrotic syndrome is the generic name for the pathological conditions associated with proteinuria (≥3.5g/day), hypoproteinemia, and generalized edema. The disorder is further classified as a

Parameter	All Subjects	Glomerulonephritis	Diabetic nephropathy	Others
Utility(QALYs)				
Mean ± SD	0.75 ± 0.21	0.73 ± 0.17	0.68 ± 0.23	0.83 ± 0.22
Median	0.73	0.71	0.60	1.00
p-value		*	**	**
Cost (USD/year)				
Mean ± SD	45,200 ± 8800	45,300 ± 8800	51,100 ± 10,700	41,100 ± 4100
Median	43,300	44,100	43,500	41,900
p-value		**	**	**
Cost-effectiveness (USD/QALY)				
Mean ± SD	68,800 ± 44,700	68,200 ± 40,700	81,700 ± 52,800	54,600 ± 27,400
Median	58,700	60,900	81,100	44,400
p-value		**	**	**
Dialysis time (hour per intervention)				
Mean ± SD		4.35 ± 0.50	4.19 ± 0.39	4.08 ± 0.43
95%CI(two-sample population mean)		0.16(0.01.0.28)	0.27(0.16, 0.37)	0.11(-0.01.0.23)
Biochemistry				
Cr(mg/dL)				
Mean ± SD		9.93 ± 2.11	9.47 ± 2.39	10.97 ± 3.24
95%CI(two-sample population mean)		0.45(-0.78, 1.70)	1.04(-0.29, 2.38)	1.50(-0.09, 3.09)
BUN(mg/dL)				
Mean ± SD		67.09 ± 15.62	69.43 ± 16.92	72.43 ± 12.38
95%CI(two-sample population mean)		2.34(-4.87, 9.56)	5.34(0.02, 10.65)	2.99(-4.20, 10.20)
Age(years)				
Mean ± SD		63.59 ± 12.30	63.78 ± 4.27	51.78 ± 14.08
95%CI(two-sample population mean)		0.18(-1.88, 2.26)	11.81(8.63, 14.99)	12.00(9.19, 14.81)

$^{*}p<0.05$. $^{**}p<0.01$. The data source for this analysis was the mean value over 4 weeks in 2011. BUN. blood urea nitrogen: CI. Confidence interval: Cr. creatinine: SD. Standard deviation: QALYs. Quality-adjusted life years. These values were analyzed by distinguishing between the primary disease of end-stage kidney disease (ESKD), glomerulonephritis, diabetic nephropathy, and others during the first 4 weeks of observation [39].

Table 2.
Cost-effectiveness by utility and cost in patients on maintenance hemodialysis (MHD).

primary nephrotic syndrome (caused by primary glomerular disease) or secondary nephrotic syndrome (caused by systemic disorders). The syndrome rapidly improves with steroid (e.g., prednisolone) and immunosuppressant (e.g., cyclosporine) treatment. Refractory cases (frequent relapse type, steroid dependence, or steroid resistance) may also occur, requiring steroid therapy for prolonged periods, for which side effects become a major issue. Therefore, there is a need for novel medical strategies to suppress relapse while reducing reliance on steroids. The regimen has not been clinically verified regarding the use of rituximab in patients with steroid-dependent nephrotic syndrome and frequently relapsing nephrotic syndrome. Still, there is a lack of evidence in health economics [42].

Therefore, we conducted a prospective clinical study of 30 patients before (with steroids and immunosuppressants) and after introducing rituximab therapy (**Figure A3**). Relapse rates and total medical expenses were selected as the primary endpoints for treatment effectiveness and treatment costs, respectively. As a secondary endpoint, cost-effectiveness was compared before and after rituximab administration in relation to previous pharmacotherapy. The observation period was 24 months before and after rituximab initiation. The authors demonstrated a statistically significant improvement in the relapse rate, from a mean of 4.30 events before administration to a mean of 0.27 events after administration. Furthermore, a significantly better prognosis emerged in the cumulative avoidance of relapse rate by Kaplan–Meier analysis ($p < 0.01$) (**Figure 13**). Finally, the total medical costs

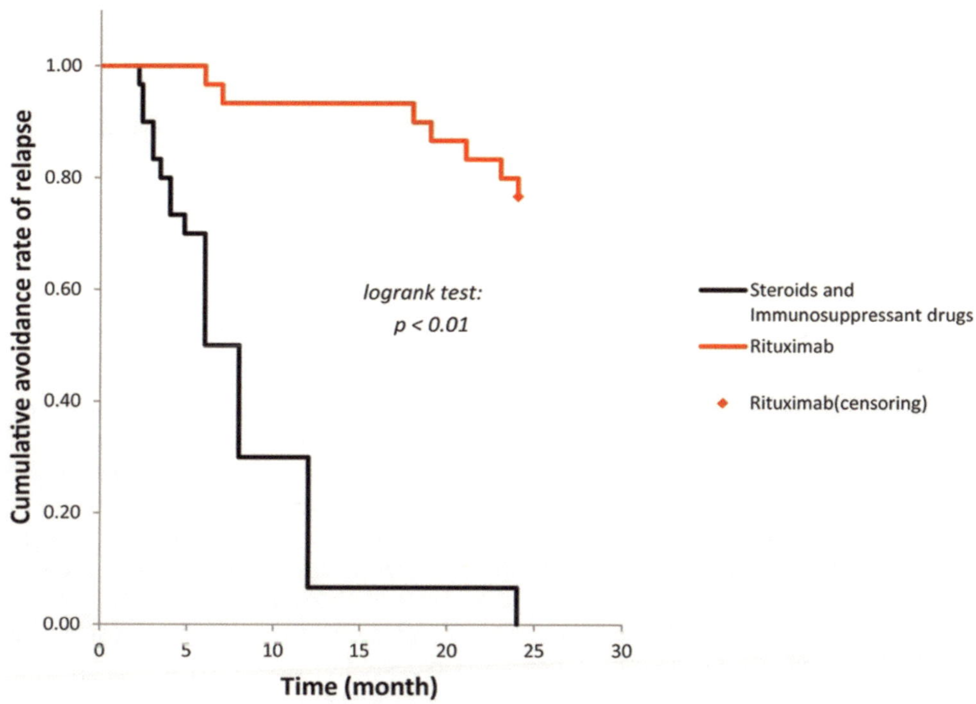

(a)

Follow up months	0	5	10	15	20	25
- Steroids and Immunosuppressant drugs (n)	30	21	9	2	2	0
- Rituximab (n)	30	30	28	28	27	24

(b)

Figure 13.
Kaplan–Meier curves of the cumulative avoidance rate of the first relapse [41].

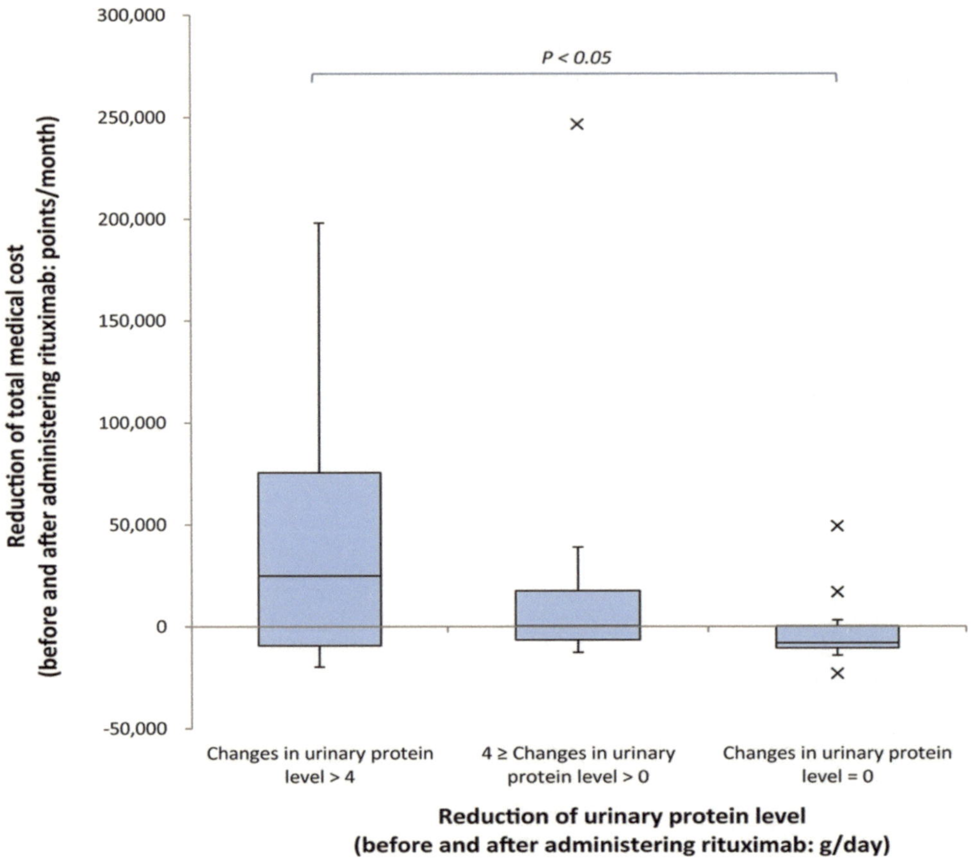

Figure 14.
Mutual relationship between urinary protein levels and total medical cost (before and after rituximab therapy) [41].

decreased from 2923 USD to 1280 USD per month, and pre-post cost-effectiveness was confirmed to be dominant (**Figure 14**). Thus, treatment with rituximab may be superior to previous pharmacological treatments from a health economics perspective (**Table 3**). Although this study did not directly observe patient utility, the excellent results in recurrence rates suggest an improvement in HRQOL.

As this study indicates the superior cost-effectiveness of rituximab against refractory nephrotic syndrome, health economics is expected to be actively applied to the valuation of technical innovations such as drug discovery.

4. Concept of price formation in the healthcare field

4.1 How to discuss price levels in the medical field

The discussion of value covers the whole range of activities related to the health and welfare field, such as examinations and diagnoses provided by medical facilities, surgery, and hospitalization, as well as medication, therapeutic materials, and care provided by caregivers. Prices (i.e., official prices in Japan) are attached to several services.

A. Exclusion of rituximab coats			
Items	Pre-administration	Post-administration	Difference (after-before)
Medical cost difference (points/ 24 months)	725,403	317,707	-407,696
(USD/24 months)	(70,155)	(30,726)	(-39,429)
Relapse difference (times/24 months)	4.30	0.27	-4.03
Pre-post CEA (points/24 months/times)			101,082
(USD/24 months/times)			(9776)
Reference: pre-post CEA with a case in which the analysis was restricted to 17 months (points/17 months/times)			50,982
(USD/17 months/times)			(4931)
B. Addition of costs for rituximab			
Items	Pre-administration	Post-administration	Difference (after-before)
Medical cost difference (points/ 24 months)	725,403	401,539	-323,864
(USD/24 months)	(70,155)	(38,833)	(-31,321)
Number of relapses (times/24 months)	4.30	0.27	-4.03
Pre-post CEA (points/24 months/times)			80,297
(USD/24 months/times)			(7766)
Reference: pre-post CEA with a case in which the analysis was restricted to 17 months (points/17 months /times)			29,445
(USD/17 months/times)			(2848)

The analysis has been corrected for the number of months. Pre-post CEA was calculated as [medical cost (post-pre)/ medical effectiveness (post-pre)] (suppression amount for medical costs accumulated over 24 months per one-time reduction[avoid] in relapses). Expressed as points per 24 months per time. Analyzing the cost-effectiveness (the ratio of total medical costs and a number of relapses, after correction for the number of months) before and after rituximab therapy revealed that cost-effectiveness improved in medical, economic terms. This was 317,707 points (30,726 USD) per 24 months (0.27 times) after rituximab therapy compared with 725,403 points (70,155 USD) per 24 months (4.30 times) before therapy [41].

Table 3.
Medical economics analysis (pre-post-CEA) accounting for the medical costs of rituximab.

Professionals who typically work in clinical or long-term care sites may not be very aware of these prices. However, the financial resources for the operation of medical and long-term care facilities are based on the price of services provided to patients/family members and long-term care recipients, who are the so-called beneficiaries. The medical institution charges to insurer for various services provided to the assured patient, which become the source of salary payments and reinvestment for the parties concerned. Therefore, if the price, value to be generated, and amount of resources consumed are not well balanced, the motivation for the employment of professionals and profitability assumedly decreases, thus making sustainable facility management difficult.

Consequently, the supply of medical and long-term care will decline, which is a significant problem for residents, including patients and their families [43–45]. Therefore, the price levels at which service recipients and providers are mutually satisfied (or convinced) should be discussed. However, determining the characteristics and effects of the target market is necessary to discuss the appropriateness of the price, considering the theory related to human choice and behavior (outlined in the previous section). In particular, as the field of health and welfare has service characteristics that are different from those in other fields, it is necessary to consider and interpret the mechanism of the market. Against this background, this section explains the basic price and its calculation methods.

The behavior and motivation of market economic agents and the pricing mechanism for goods and services, including resource allocation and income distribution, should be considered for price optimization. Overall, the general economic approach is limited because of various uncertainties related to highly specialized technologies in medical science. Thus, examining price settings in the medical field is generally difficult because of the complex involvement of various factors. A price-setting approach in medical treatment can be divided into two major categories: "market-based" and "input-based" [46]. The "market-based" approach determines the price level by considering the actual market price of medical treatment, while the "input-based" approach is based on the consumption of goods and services. Generally, prices are presumed to have been formed in the public medical market using these approaches in countries with a mature medical system.

Approaches to explain the public price of individual medical technologies (services) have also been discussed. For example, from the standpoint of a medical provider (supply approach), "technical difficulty" and "medical cost" are often selected from the viewpoint of quality evaluation and business management. Furthermore, for the payer (or beneficiary), the methods of "patient outcome," "economic performance," and "willingness to pay" are often selected from the perspective of market and value evaluation (**Figure 15**) [48–50]. Additionally, cases exist in which certain preconditions are set to use these indicators. For example, in Japan's universal health insurance system, most prices charged to public insurers by medical institutions are centered on direct

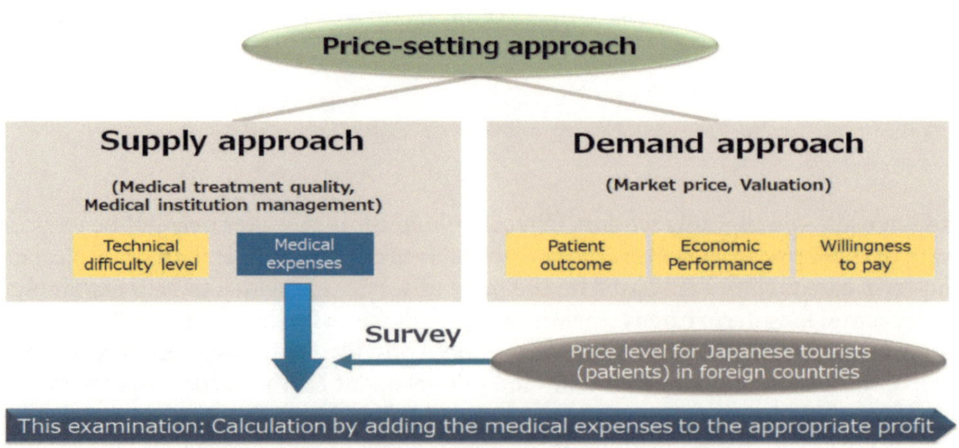

Figure 15.
Theory of the price-setting approach (in general and within the range of this examination) [47].

medical costs, based on the consumption of medical resources—considering their clinical usefulness and hospital operability. Technical fees (e.g., surgery fees), influenced by doctors' specialties, are considered technical difficulties. Furthermore, overseas (developed countries) market prices are referred to when determining the public prices for pharmaceutical resources and medical devices.

As the socio-economic environment surrounding the medical system becomes more severe, even public prices that follow the theory of the public economy are expected to play a role in improving the system's performance and increasing its sustainability. In other words, verifying the structure of price formation and the appropriateness of its level has become a major concern for medical stakeholders. Based on this, an analysis of factors that affect prices is also expected. However, when developing official price research in the medical field, the following must be noted: There are not enough research reports to study the analytical model required for factor analysis. This condition is especially true in Japan. In addition, the formation of official prices involves various subsidy programs (politics), and thus, the analytical approach becomes too complicated. Therefore, in this chapter, as an initial study on medical prices, we introduce a survey on price differences between Japan and overseas and price factors in the private market.

This study examines the mechanism of market price reference and the influence of the real economy (citizens' economic burden) on the public price, contributing to the arrangement of public price discussions in the future.

4.2 Research example of medical pricing for foreigners visiting Japan

This section presents a method for setting the price level based on the analysis of medical expenses of Japanese medical institutions for foreign visitors (FVs). Furthermore, international comparisons of price levels for Japanese tourists (patients) in foreign countries have been conducted previously [47]. This section elucidates the "market-based" and "input-based" approaches discussed in 4.1, and discusses the "foreign price reference system," which is part of the setting of public prices in Japan. In recent years, the supply of medical services centered on pharmaceutical products has been based on global R&D, manufacturing, and sales systems. In addition, some patient groups also exhibit cross-border consultation behaviors. In other words, it is inferred that discussions with a view to the globalization of medical care are indispensable for the progress of UHC, even if they are indirect.

The costs were analyzed based on socio-economic ranges in this calculation, considering clinical characteristics and economic activities. The costs related to general medical care and public investment in hospital management and healthcare infrastructure through the insurance system and various taxation systems that support Japan's medical system are also considered. For example, social insurance burdens (e.g., insurance contributions and subsidies, such as operational grants to medical institutions) and additional expenses for FVs (e.g., interpretation, coordinator, equipment, and risk management costs) were used as calculation items.

Three medical institutions with more than 400 beds were chosen as target facilities, and their locations (urban or rural) were considered. Additional factors (such as the occupancy and profit rate of each facility) were considered in the calculation. Data collection involved medical practice and medical institution management surveys. The medical practice survey used time study (i.e., occupation time of medical staff and institutional equipment) and medical records (i.e., electronic and management ledgers): Some were self-reported alternatives based on their professional experience.

The medical institution management survey collected financial statements (profit and loss balance sheets), number of patients and medical treatments, number of staff and equipment, unit purchase price, and the area of each department.

The medical expenses for FVs were broadly divided into "additional expenses of foreign medical treatment" and "increased expenses of regular medical treatment." The following definitions for additional and increased expenses were applied: additional expenses for new and additional services (e.g., interpretation and transportation) for non-locally insured patients. The increased expenses for medical services were similarly offered to the locally-insured patients. However, for non-locally-insured patients, the unit price and quantity increased (e.g., consultation hours and staff). Profit was included in this calculation as a necessary resource for reinvestment by medical institutions to realize sustainable management while appropriately responding to the medical needs of FVs. However, when determining profit margins, the historical average of each institution was adopted to avoid the distortion of price levels and the expensive economic burden on FVs owing to excessive profits. The profits gained from FVs were essentially the same as those from Japanese patients.

Compared with the medical expenses (point system) of Japanese patients, those for FVs were 1.31 times (1 point 0.12 dollars) higher for pharyngitis, 1.56 times (1 point 0.14 dollars) higher for urticaria with allergies, 2.21 times (1 point 0.20 dollars) higher for hemorrhagic cystitis, 3.66 times (1 point 0.34 dollars) higher for in patients with severe pneumonia, 1.22 times (1 point 0.11 dollars) higher for general appendicitis, and 2.92 times (1 point 0.27 dollars) higher for endoscopic cholangitis treatment (**Figure 16**). Moreover, the operating expense for trochanteric fractures of the femur was 3.59 times (1 point 0.33 dollars) higher. **Figure 17** shows the amount billed when providing medical treatment to Japanese overseas travelers (overseas FVs) in each country. The survey indicated that although the total number of patients was 18 (one in each country, except for the USA, Australia, Italy, and China), the actual medical payment was approximately USD 20.32–158.75/bill (medical expenditures for medical examination and drug cost) in 12 countries. The highest price was in the USA, at USD 158.75/bill (medical fees may be partially unknown), followed by Austria with USD 79.38 (purchasing power parity 86.28)/bill and Belgium with USD 73.93 (purchasing power parity 73.93)/bill. In summary, including additional research, the medical expenses for FV patients were 1.22–3.66 times higher than those for Japanese patients,

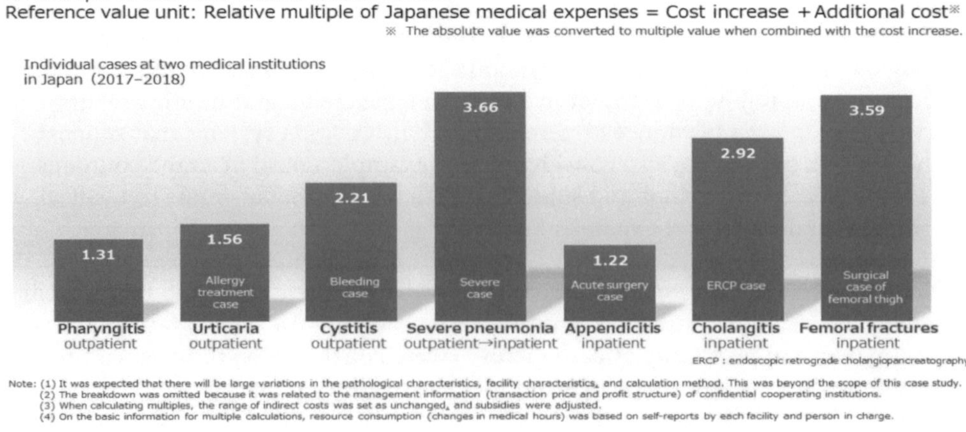

Figure 16.
Calculation of price levels for foreign visitors (seven diseases) [47].

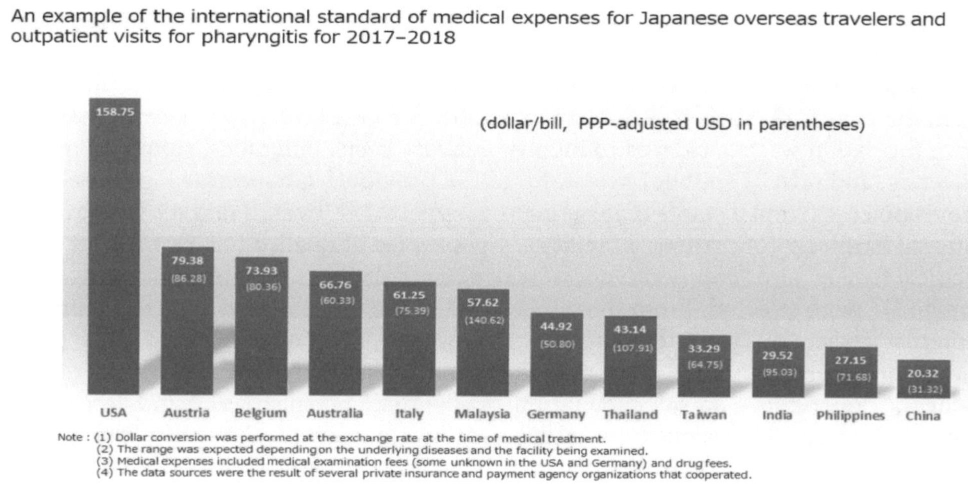

Figure 17.
International comparison of medical expenses (pharyngitis and outpatients) [47].

1.31–2.21 times higher for outpatients (pharyngitis, urticaria, and cystitis), and 1.22–3.66 times higher for inpatients (e.g., with severe pneumonia, appendicitis, cholangitis, and femoral fractures).

4.3 Examples of studies related to factors that form the parturition price

The concept of factors that form the parturition price operated by the private medical care system (out-of-pocket) and the actual situation of the difference in price level due to regional characteristics [51] is introduced. This approach spans both "market-based" and "input-based" approaches, as discussed in Section 4.1. For the sustainable operation of the medical system, it is important to consider the stability of hospital management and the financial burden on citizens. In other words, it is presumed that discussions that consider the relationship between economic factors and medical treatment behavior are indispensable for the progress of UHC. This study has the advantage of developing purely causal inferences on that subject, considering the bias of other social support (subsidies). It is useful to indirectly re-recognize how the ratio of out-of-pocket expenses to the official price of public medical insurance affects the choice of consultation.

In Japan, parturition (normal childbirth), which differs from injury and illness, is not covered by the medical insurance system. This service is self-financed medical care. However, as financial support for childbirth expenditures, the Health Insurance Act provides a lump-sum childbirth and childcare allowance of JPY 420,000 per child (2021). As this system aims to reduce the financial burden of childbirth, it is also important from the perspective of measures against declining birth rates. However, the average price of childbirth is rising, and the actual cost of childbirth often exceeds JPY 420,000. Therefore, while an increase in the amount of lump-sum childbirth and childcare payments has been requested, the out-of-pocket price structure of childbirth is unclear; that is, actual costs have not been understood. Therefore, the government considers the appropriate amount of lump-sum childbirth and childcare payments to realistically grasp the situation of childbirth expenditures with services and prices.

Against the background of these trends, Japan's regional levels of parturition prices and the factors that helped inform them were analyzed. First, a hypothesis that market principles would have a greater effect on the level formation was proposed; then, the factors that affect childbirth expenditures were structured. Consequently, price formation was considered to involve delivery costs, outcomes, supply/demand, solvency, and official (public) prices. From the provider's perspective, "guarantee of provision cost (from a stable management viewpoint)," "overall market level and internal harmony (operation of facility)," "guarantee of quality (characteristics of the medical field)," and "competitiveness of regions (balance between supply and demand)" were selected. From the perspective of pregnant women, the elements of "interest in security (from the outcome perspective)," "interest in added value (from the amenity perspective)," "interest in the brand (from the perspective of other added values)," "restrictions on solvency (from an economic perspective)," and "access conditions (from the various types of burden)" were selected. Generally, childbirth expenditure is affected by various factors, including different factors related to facility type (e.g., general hospital, clinic, and maternity home), delivery method (e.g., natural childbirth, cesarean section, and painless delivery), timing (weekdays/daytime, night/holidays, year-end/new year), region (prefectures, cities/regions), and others (e.g., optional services such as attending a birth with family).

Consequently, the average parturition price by region in Japan was investigated. First, when the actual situation of childbirth expenditure by prefecture was analyzed using national birth-related statistical data (around 2016) [52, 53], the national average was 505,759 ± 41,906 JPY/case. A difference of approximately 1.5 times was confirmed between the highest (Tokyo City: No.1 in **Figure 18**) and lowest (Tottori Prefecture: No.48 in **Figure 18**) areas. Subsequently, multivariate analysis (multiple regression analysis) was performed to analyze the factors that differed depending on regional characteristics. Based on the factor structure described above, the objective variable was the parturition price. The explanatory variables were citizen income (solvency), "public medical expense (hospitalization unit price)," "pregnant woman's

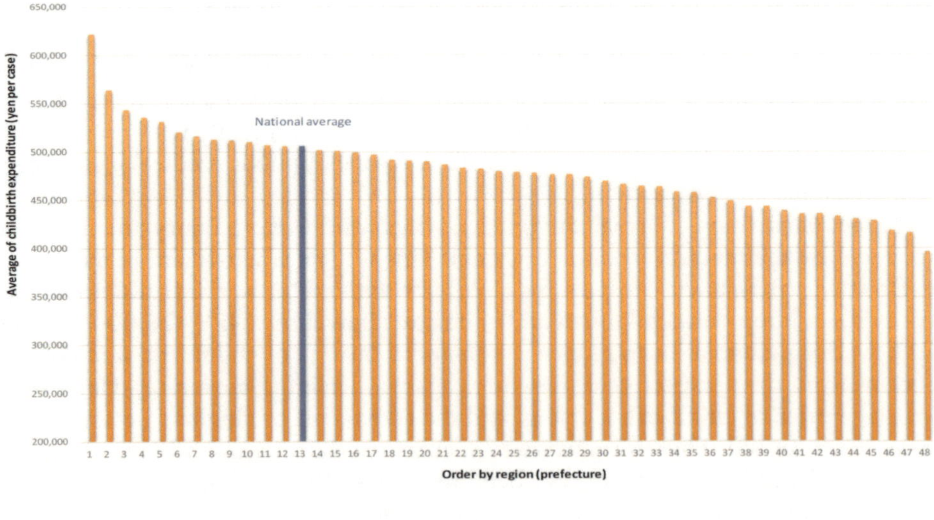

Figure 18.
Distribution of parturition prices by region (prefecture). Note: The data source was "mean and median of childbirth costs by prefecture" (All-Japan Federation of National Health Insurance Organizations, announced in 2017).

Childbirth expenditures (normal childbirth, yen / case, FY2016)	Standardized partial regression coefficient	F-value	p-value	VIF
Annual income per citizen of the prefecture (yen / year)	0.561	17.588	0.000**	2.68
1-day hospitalization unit public price for all beds (overall: yen / day)	0.281	4.106	0.054	2.88
Pregnant woman age (years)	0.331	4.384	0.047*	3.74
Total number of births (cases)	−0.628	7.011	0.014*	8.42
Average number of births per hospital facility (number of deliveries: cases)	0.312	3.272	0.083	4.46
Maternal and fetal intensive care unit per birth population (MFICU: number of beds)	−0.257	5.162	0.032*	1.91
Decentralized analysis of the model: $p < 0.001$				
*: $p < 0.05$, **: $p < 0.01$				

Note: MFICU, maternal-fetal intensive care unit.

Table 4.
Socio-economic factors are affecting parturition price levels (multiple regression analysis).

age (risk factor)," "birth population (childbirth demand)," and "obstetric facility (supply capacity)," and "specialized equipment (maternal-fetal intensive care unit). The statistical software SPSS (IBM) was used for analysis, and the significance level was set at 5%. The results indicate that prefectural income, age at parturition, number of births, and density of equipment (facilities) affect parturition prices (**Table 4**). In particular, the citizen income (standard partial regression coefficient: 0.561, $p < 0.001$) tended to be highly related to parturition prices. The standard partial regression coefficient of birth population was negative (−0.628, $p = 0.014$), but the simple regression coefficient was positive (0.721, $p < 0.01$).

5. Conclusion

This chapter discussed the macroscopic mechanisms of the relationship between UHC progress and socio-economic factors to promote the sustainable development of health insurance systems. Against that background, the clinical economic considerations were presented to discuss the relationship between value and price from a micro perspective (e.g., health technology assessment).

Examining the effects of socio-economic factors of GDP and governmental health expenditures on the development of UHC showed a statistically significant positive correlation between these factors and UHC service coverage index. Furthermore, it was understood that the declining birth rate, aging population, and maturing healthcare system impacted the progress of UHC. Unemployment and poverty, distant causes of catastrophic healthcare costs, reduced the service coverage index level because of the mechanisms related to vital statistics and economic conditions. Thus, policymakers must implement countermeasures based on indicators that can estimate the economic status of the UHC approach, such as its cost-effectiveness. The sufficiency of public healthcare resources was considered important in addressing this issue. Furthermore, it was inferred that sharing healthcare values among stakeholders would be meaningful for this purpose.

Assuming that it contributes to the discussion of the real economy and official prices related to the medical field, the medical value should be evaluated by applying the marginal utility theory and cost-utility analysis. Despite some limitations, the benefits and burdens based on the value of medical care should be discussed when designing a system related to the operation of medical insurance. In this chapter, valuation research cases related to the significance of lifesaving and drug discovery were introduced, considering the possibility of allocating public resources. Furthermore, present chapter presented the price formation mechanism in the clinical field based on medical value. The price level was organized with reference to the case (childbirth) of private medical care in Japan. Factors such as the age at parturition, income level, and facility utilization rate have a price impact.

Promoting harmonization with socio-economic trends and improving explanatory power for those who bear the economic burden are key points for the future development of medical insurance systems. Long-term research using a broader range of socio-economic indicators is needed for a more accurate interpretation and deeper analysis of the obtained findings.

Acknowledgements

This study was funded by the Government of Japan Health and Labor Sciences Research Grant (grant no. JP19DA1004).

Conflict of interest

The author declares no conflicts of interest associated with this manuscript.

Notes/thanks/other declarations

The authors gratefully acknowledge Ms. Naoko Tsukamoto and Ms. Noriko Yoshida for their contributions to the chart adjustment.

A. Appendix

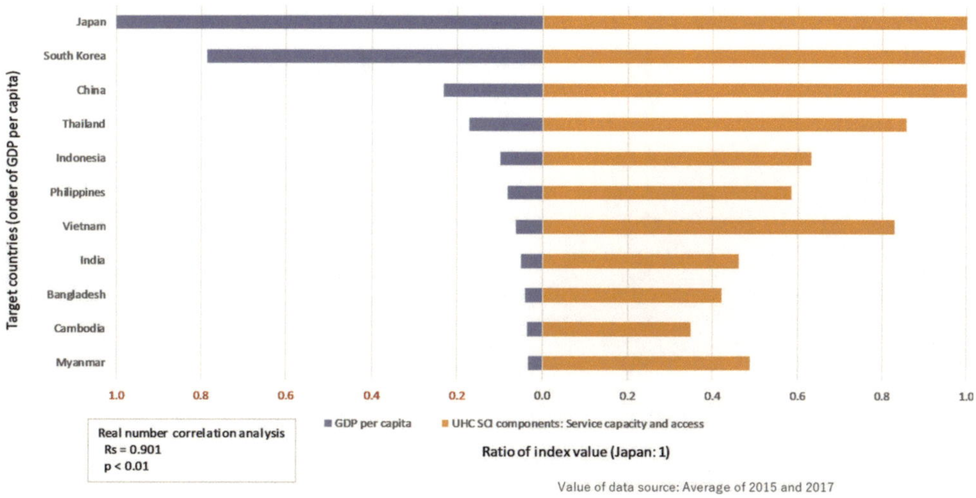

Figure A1.
Trends in the country-specific economic level (GDP) and SCI components (service capacity and access). Note: UHC, universal health coverage; SCI, service coverage index [21].

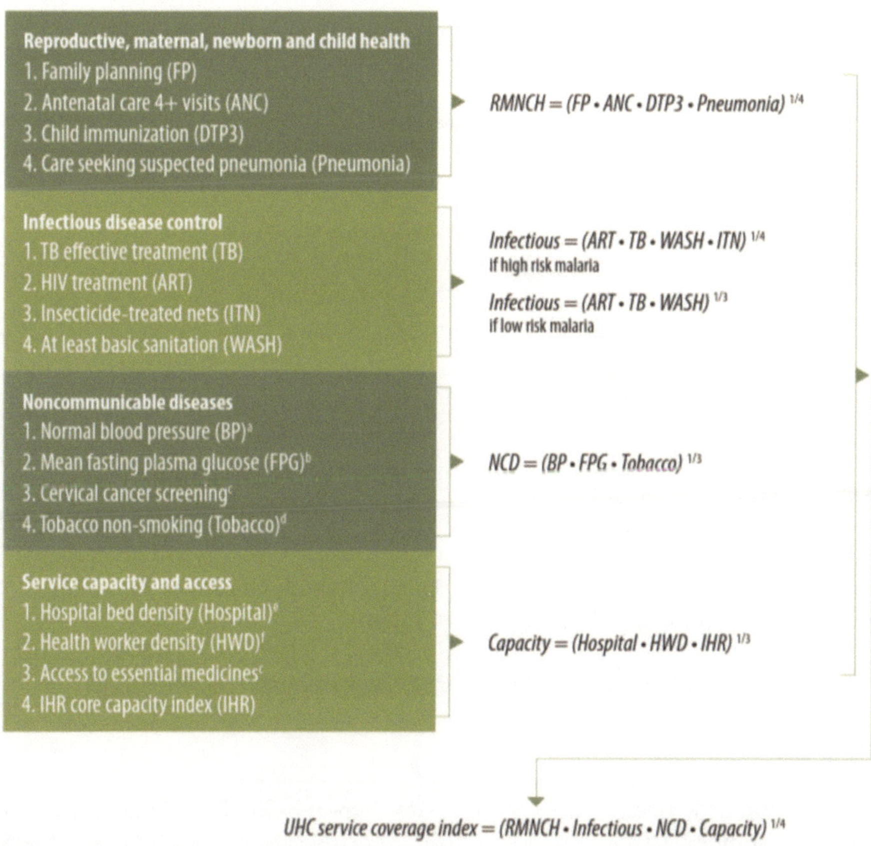

Figure A2.
The UHC service coverage index (SCI): Summary of tracer indicators and computation [4].

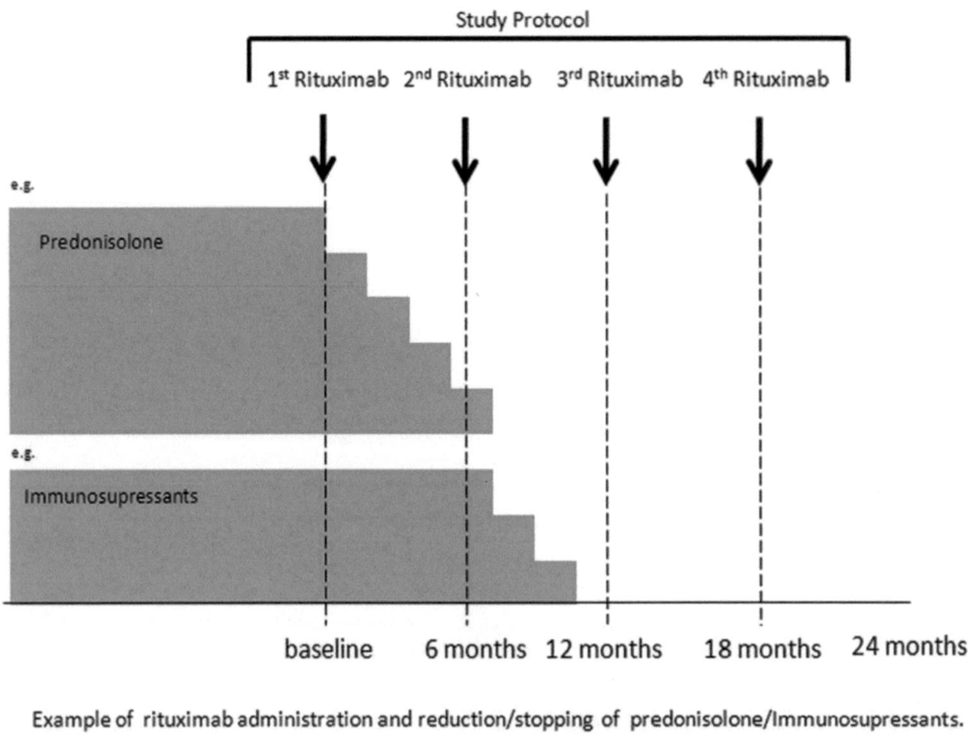

Figure A3.
Overview of the regimen used (images). In this study, rituximab was administered four times every 6 months. For the first 6 months after the first dose of rituximab, the dosage of prednisolone and cyclosporine was reduced each month and stopped [41].

Author details

Tomoyuki Takura
Department of Healthcare Economics and Health Policy, Graduate School of Medicine, The University of Tokyo, Tokyo, Japan

*Address all correspondence to: ttakura@m.u-tokyo.ac.jp

References

[1] Tambor M, Klich J, Domagała A. Financing healthcare in central and eastern European countries: How far are we from universal health coverage? International Journal of Environmental Research and Public Health. 2021;**18**(4): 1382. DOI: 10.3390/ijerph18041382

[2] Takura T. An evaluation of clinical economics and case of cost-effectiveness. Internal Medicine. 2018; **57**(9):1191-1200. DOI: 10.2169/internalmedicine.9835-17

[3] Sen A. Collective Choice and Social Welfare; an Expanded Edition. London: Harvard University Press; 2018. p. 640

[4] World Health Organization. Tracking Universal Health Coverage. Global Monitoring Report [Internet]. 2017. [cited 2021-08-22]. Available from: https://apps.who.int/iris/bitstream/handle/10665/259817/9789241513555-eng.pdf

[5] Cleemput I, Kesteloot K, DeGeest S. A review of the literature on the economics of noncompliance. Room for methodological improvement. Health Policy. 2002;**59**(1):65-94

[6] Robertson CT, Yuan A, Zhang W, Joiner K. Distinguishing moral hazard from access for high-cost healthcare under insurance. PLoS One. 2020;**15**(4): e0231768. DOI: 10.1371/journal.pone.0231768

[7] Hassanally K. Overgrazing in general practice: The new tragedy of the commons. The British Journal of General Practice. 2015;**65**(631):81. DOI: 10.3399/bjgp15X683581

[8] Porco TC, Daozhou G, Scott JC, Shim E, Enanoria WT, Galvani AP, et al. When does overuse of antibiotics become a tragedy of the commons? PLoS One. 2012;**7**(12):e46505. DOI: 10.1371/journal.pone.0046505

[9] McIntyre D, Thiede M, Dahlgren G, Whitehead M. What are the economic consequences for households of illness and of paying for health care in low- and middle-income country contexts? Social Science & Medicine. 2006;**62**(4):858-865. DOI: 10.1016/j.socscimed.2005.07.001

[10] Stepurko T, Pavlova M, Groot W. Overall satisfaction of health care users with the quality of and access to health care services: A cross-sectional study in six central and eastern European countries. BMC Health Services Research. 2016;**16**(a):342. DOI: 10.1186/s12913-016-1585-1

[11] Zink A, Rose S. Fair regression for health care spending. Biometrics. 2020; **76**(3):973-982. DOI: 10.1111/biom.13206

[12] McGuire TG, Schillo S, van Kleef RC. Very high and low residual spenders in private health insurance markets: Germany, the Netherlands, and the US marketplaces. The European Journal of Health Economics. 2021;**22**(1):35-50. DOI: 10.1007/s10198-020-01227-3

[13] Patcharanarumol W, Panichkriangkrai W, Sommanuttaweechai A, Hanson K, Wanwong Y, Tangcharoensathien V. Strategic purchasing and health system efficiency: A comparison of two financing schemes in Thailand. PLoS One. 2018;**13**(4):e0195179. DOI: 10.1371/journal.pone.0195179

[14] Kroneman M, Boerma W, van den Berg M, Groenewegen P, de Jong J, van Ginneken E. Netherlands: Health System Review. Health Systems in Transition. Netherlands: Health Communications. 2016;18(2):1-240.

[15] Kreng VB, Yang CT. The equality of resource allocation in health care under the National Health Insurance System in Taiwan. Health Policy. 2011;**100**(2–3): 203-210. DOI: 10.1016/j.healthpol. 2010.08.003

[16] Saultz JW, Jones SM, McDaniel SH, Bagley B, McCormally T, Marker JE, et al. A new foundation for the delivery and financing of American Health Care. Family Medicine. 2015;**47**(8): 612-619

[17] World Health Organization. Universal health coverage [Internet]; 2021. [cited 2021-08-22]. Available from: https://www.who.int/westernpacific/health-topics/universal-health-coverag

[18] World Health Organization. Monitoring report [Internet]; 2019. [cited 2021-08-22]. Available from: http://www.who.int/healthinfo/universal_health_coverage/report/2019/en/

[19] Laranjeira E, Szrek H. Going beyond life expectancy in assessments of health systems' performance: Life expectancy adjusted by perceived health status. International Journal of Health Economics and Management. 2016; **16**(2):133-161. DOI: 10.1007/s10754-015-9183-z

[20] Moon S, Shin J. Performance of universal health insurance: Lessons from South Korea. World Health & Population. 2007;**9**(2):95-113. DOI: 10.12927/whp.2007.18882

[21] Takura T, Miura H. Socioeconomic determinants of universal health coverage in the Asian region. International Journal of Environmental Research and Public Health. 2022;**19**(4): 2376. DOI: 10.3390/ijerph19042376

[22] Rao KD, Makimoto S, Peters M, et al. Vulnerable populations, and universal health coverage. In: Kharas H, McArthur JW, Ohno I, editors. Leave No One behind: Time for Specifics on the Sustainable Development Goals. Washington, DC: Brookings Institution Press; 2019. pp. 129-148

[23] UHC. Core content for understanding UHC and public health budgets [Internet]; 2021. [cited 2021-08-22]. Available from: https://www.uhc2030.org/what-we-do/voices/accountability/budget-toolkit/chapter-2-core-content-for-understanding-uhc-and-public-budgets-for-health/

[24] Eregata GT, Hailu A, Memirie ST, Norheim OF. Measuring progress towards universal health coverage: National and subnational analysis in Ethiopia. BMJ Global Health. 2019;**4**(6): e001843. DOI: 10.1136/bmjgh-2019-001843

[25] Sasaki T, Izawa M, Okada Y. Current trends in health insurance systems: OECD countries vs Japan. Neurologia Medico-Chirurgica. 2015;**55**(4):267-275. DOI: 10.2176/nmc.ra.2014-0317

[26] GBD Universal health coverage collaborators. Measuring universal health coverage based on an index of effective coverage of health services in 204 countries and territories, 1990–2019: A systematic analysis for the global burden of disease study. Open Access Published. 2019;**2020**. DOI: 10.1016/S0140-6736(20)30750-9

[27] The World Bank Group. World Bank open data. 2021. [cited 22 Oct 2021]. Available from: https://data.worldbank.org

[28] World Health Organization. UHC index of service coverage (SCI). 2021. [cited 22 Oct 2021]. Available from:

https://www.who.int/data/gho/data/indicators/indicator-details/GHO/uhc-index-of-service-coverage

[29] World Health Organization. Global Health, Observatory. 2022. [cited 22 Jun 2021]. Available from: https://www.who.int/data/gho

[30] Global Burden of Disease Health Financing Collaborator Network. Trends in future health financing and coverage: Future health spending and universal health coverage in 188 countries, 2016-40. Lancet. 2018;**391**(10132): 1783-1798

[31] Musgrove P. Cost-effectiveness and the socialization of health care. Health Policy. 1995;**32**(1–3):111-123. DOI: 10.1016/0168-8510(95)00730-g

[32] Dean E, Elardo J, Green M, Wilson B, Berger S. Principles of Microeconomics: Scarcity and Social Provisioning. Oregon: Open Oregon Educational Resources; 2020. p. 821. Available from: https://openoregon.pressbooks.pub/socialprovisioning/

[33] Ottolini FL, Buggio L, Somigliana E, Vercellini P. The complex interface between economy and healthcare: An introductory overview for clinicians. European Journal of Internal Medicine. 2016;**36**:1-6. DOI: 10.1016/j.ejim.2016.07.030

[34] Principles of Economics. Vol. 1236. Minneapolis: University of Minnesota libraries publishing; 2016. DOI: 10.24926/8668.1601

[35] Takura T. Value and Price of Medicine- toward the Age of Choice and Decision. Tokyo: Igaku-Shoin; 2021. p. 276

[36] Ibe T, Kanai M, Takura T, et al. Nursing management learning text. In: Management Resource Management Theory. 3rd ed. Tokyo: Japanese Nursing Association; 2020. p. 304

[37] Mitchell RC, Carson RT. Using Surveys to Value Public Goods. Vol. 484. Washington DC: Resources for the Future; 1989. DOI: 10.2307/2072944

[38] Takura T. Contact lens medical care and health economics. Journal of Japanese Contact Lens Society. 2009; **51**(3):204-209

[39] Takura T, Nakanishi T, Kawanishi H, Nitta K, Akizawa T, Hiramatsu M, et al. Cost-effectiveness of maintenance hemodialysis in Japan. Therapeutic Apheresis and Dialysis. 2015;**19**(5):441-449. DOI: 10.1111/1744-9987.12314

[40] Liyanage T, Toyama T, Hockham C, Ninomiya T, Perkovic V, Woodward M, et al. Prevalence of chronic kidney disease in Asia: A systematic review and analysis. BMJ Global Health. 2022;**7**(1): e007525. DOI: 10.1136/bmjgh-2021-007525

[41] Takura T, Takei T, Nitta K. Cost-effectiveness of rituximab administration for steroid-dependent nephrotic syndrome and frequently relapsing nephrotic syndrome: A preliminary study in Japan. Scientific Reports. 2017;**7**:46036. DOI: 10.1038/srep46036

[42] Bruchfeld A, Benedek S, Hilderman M, Medin C, Snaedal-Jonsdottir S, Korkeila M. Rituximab for minimal change disease in adults: Long-term follow-up. Nephrology, Dialysis, Transplantation. 2014;**29**(4):851-856

[43] Japan Tourism Organization. Monthly/Yearly Statistical Data (Foreign Visitors/Japanese Departures). Tokyo, Japan: Japan Tourism Organization; 2018

[44] Ministry of Health, Labour and Welfare health insurance in Japan. Survey on the acceptance of foreign patients at medical institutions [Internet]. 2018. [cited 2021-04-30]. Available from: https://www.mhlw.go.jp/stf/seisakunitsuite/bunya/0000202918_00014.html

[45] Ministry of Health, Labour and Welfare health insurance in Japan [Internet]. [cited 2021-02-28]. Available from: https://www.mhlw.go.jp/stf/seisakunitsuite/bunya/kenkou_iryou/iryouhoken/iryouhoken01/index.html

[46] Smith SL, Gallagher PE. Medicare RBRVS 1997: The Physicians Guide. Chicago, IL: American Medical Association; 1997

[47] Takura T. Study group research on appropriate medical treatment prices for foreigners visiting Japan. Preliminary examination of an appropriate price calculation method and medical treatment costs for foreign visitors in Japan. International Journal of Environmental Research and Public Health. 2021;**18**(11): 5837. DOI: 10.3390/ijerph18115837

[48] Hsiao WC, Braun P, Dunn DL, Becker ER, Yntema D, Verrilli DK, et al. An overview of the development and refinement of the resource-based relative value scale: The foundation for reform of US physician payment. Medical Care. 1992;**30**(Suppl. 1): NS1-NS12

[49] Miller FA, Lehoux P, Peacock S, Rac VE, Neukomm J, Barg C, et al. How procurement judges the value of medical technologies: A review of healthcare tenders. International Journal of Technology Assessment in Health Care. 2019;**35**(1):50-55

[50] Morrisey MA. Hospital pricing: Cost shifting and competition. EBRI Issue Brief. 1993;**137**(137):1-17

[51] Takura T. Concept of childbirth cost (price level). Second Parliamentary Union to reduce the burden of childbirth expenditures. Tokyo (first members' office building of the House of Representatives). 2021. Available from: http://www.jihsr.com/member/pdf/takura/number01_24/24-1.pdf

[52] Cabinet Office of Japan. Prefectural economic calculation [Internet]. 2016. [cited 2021-08-22]. Available from: https://www.esri.cao.go.jp/jp/sna/sonota/kenmin/kenmin_top.html

[53] All-Japan Federation of National Health Insurance Organizations. Childbirth expenditures [Internet]. 2017. [cited 2021-08-22]. Available from: https://www.kokuho.or.jp/statistics/birth/2017-0620.html